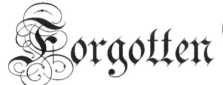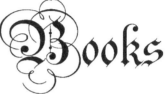
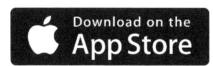
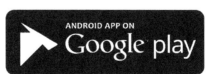

ISBN 978-0-282-53275-8
PIBN 10855421

1 MONTH OF
FREE
READING

at

www.ForgottenBooks.com

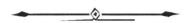

By purchasing this book you are eligible for one month membership to ForgottenBooks.com, giving you unlimited access to our entire collection of over 700,000 titles via our web site and mobile apps.

To claim your free month visit:

www.forgottenbooks.com/free855421

English
Français
Deutsche
Italiano
Español
Português

www.forgottenbooks.com

Mythology Photography **Fiction**
Fishing Christianity **Art** Cooking
Essays Buddhism Freemasonry
Medicine **Biology** Music **Ancient Egypt** Evolution Carpentry Physics
Dance Geology **Mathematics** Fitness
Shakespeare **Folklore** Yoga Marketing
Confidence Immortality Biographies
Poetry **Psychology** Witchcraft
Electronics Chemistry History **Law**
Accounting **Philosophy** Anthropology
Alchemy Drama Quantum Mechanics
Atheism Sexual Health **Ancient History**
Entrepreneurship Languages Sport
Paleontology Needlework Islam
Metaphysics Investment Archaeology
Parenting Statistics Criminology
Motivational

FUNDAMENTAL GYMNASTICS

The Basis of Rational Physical Development

BY

NIELS BUKH

Principal, Gymnastic Peoples College, Ollerup, Denmark
Author of "PRIMARY GYMNASTICS," etc.

Translated from the second Danish edition, rearranged
and adapted for use in America

BY

EMILY RUSSELL ANDREWS

Instructor in the theory and practice of gymnastics and self-
testing activities; Central School of Hygiene and Physical
Education, New York City; Instructor in theory
of Fundamental Gymnastics, American Sum-
mer Courses, Ollerup, Denmark

AND

KAREN VESTERDAL

Formerly, Assistant Instructor in gymnastics and folk dancing;
Central School of Hygiene and Physical Education,
New York City; Instructor of Song Games, Amer-
ican Summer Courses, Ollerup, Denmark

WITH MANY NEW ILLUSTRATIONS

E. P. DUTTON AND COMPANY

PUBLISHERS   NEW YORK

FIRST EDITION

FOREWORD

My wish for the American edition of this book is that it may prove of value to teachers who are interested in building a strong and practical foundation for the *P*hysical Education of the American youth.

Athletics, ball playing, swimming, games and dancing are excellent mediums for use in the education of the people but these activities are effective and productive of good results in proportion as the body is able to execute them with efficiency and beauty.

Gymnastics are fundamental to sports and they must remain so. Through gymnastics, the body may be so perfectly moulded, strengthened and co-ordinated that the youth is never conscious of it as a hindrance, or as incapable of achieving for him anything he may be ambitious to do. On the contrary, the possession of a perfectly co-ordinating bodily mechanism proves the greatest stimulus to youth to enter into all sports and test his power.

When through gymnastic work the body has been made beautiful and efficient, and youth is irresistibly drawn to sports and activities of all kinds, then can *P*hysical Education realize, through these, its highest and ultimate aims in the development of character and personality.

NIELS BUKH

PREFACE

The Gymnastic *P*eoples College in Ollerup, Denmark, is one of the representative institutions of the great movement for adult education in which Denmark is leading the world. These schools give an opportunity for continued study which is eagerly embraced by the young men and women of the rural communities. Young men attend the schools from November to April, when there is little work to be done on the farms, and the girls are in session from May through July.

All the *P*eoples Colleges include gymnastics in their curriculum but Niels Bukh's school in Ollerup is the only one that specializes in this subject. The course of study is similar to those of the other *P*eoples Colleges, including geography, history, mathematics, language and religion but has the added subjects of physiology, anatomy, theory of teaching, gymnastics, ball games and folk dancing necessary in a school of this type.

After graduation from Mr. Bukh's school, the boys and girls go back to their home communities as volunteer leaders, but they are not recognized as trained teachers of physical education until they have taken the one year course in the States Institute in Copenhagen.

A little more than ten years ago Niels Bukh, then a teacher of physical education in one of the *P*eoples Colleges, became dissatisfied with the results of his use of Swedish gymnastics in correcting the maladjustments and faulty occupational habits of posture and carriage of his students. With a small group of boys he began experimenting with exercises which were freer in style, contained a wider range of movement, and were more organically stimulating.

His success was immediate and dramatic and he was asked to demonstrate his type of work in many parts of Denmark and Sweden. Wherever his work was shown it met with the delighted acceptance of youth, but with criticism and censure from the leaders of gymnastics who saw no legitimate place in the educational scheme for exercises not traditionally Swedish. With belief in his work, and the goal ever before him of a "steadfast, beautiful youth," he worked quietly, unperturbed by hardship and unpopularity until he stands today acknowledged as one of the foremost leaders of Danish youth.

There are still many people in Denmark who, for personal or political reasons, do not agree with his principles and methods, but the work is rapidly and profoundly influencing the gymnastics taught in the schools, and it has been recently adopted by the Danish army. Teachers from all parts of the world have visited Ollerup and many have remained to take the course. Eager exponents have carried the work to enthusiastic recipients in England, Iceland, Germany, Holland, Finland, Belgium, Turkey, Austria-Hungary, Czecho-Slovakia and the United States. Mr. Bukh has been invited to give many demonstrations throughout central Europe and has everywhere been greeted with warm acclaim. His book, "Grundgymnastik," has been translated into nine languages and over 70,000 copies have been sold in Germany alone. At a conference in Germany in 1922, one of the foremost German educators pronounced the work shown by Mr. Bukh's students as of more value than all that the Germans had themselves been exhibiting. This statement was received at that time with great opposition, but the Germans have of late been sending their teachers in large numbers as students to both the winter and special summer courses.

Mr. Bukh's original book was written as a syllabus to accompany the lectures and practical instruction given to his students at Ollerup. It is, therefore, obviously lacking in much of the technical theory which the student and teacher of physical education expects to find in a teaching manual.

To those who make a study of the work there is no lack of sound and fundamental theory. I have been a student in Ollerup for two summers and have discussed all phases of the work in detail with Mr. Bukh. He comments humorously but regretfully on the many people who visit his classes but are so busy writing down exercises that they have no time to question him regarding the aims and values of the work, and go away with no conception or understanding of his theories. When he speaks of the few people who, with such superficial knowledge, write of and teach his work, as exponents of his theory and principles, there is deep indignation in his voice and manner and no recognition of such self-alleged friends.

Karen Vesterdal is one of Mr. Bukh's most intelligent and skillful students and has taken three courses at the school. She is a graduate of the States Institute in Copenhagen, has taught Mr. Bukh's work in Denmark, and was for two years an instructor at the Central School in New York. Her intimate knowledge of the work and of its application to American use, led Mr. Bukh to consider her pre-eminently fitted to assist in the preparation of an American edition of his book. It is at his request that Miss Vesterdal and I have undertaken the task of compiling such a text and of making such necessary changes as we feel are important in adapting it to the teaching situation in the United States. Our keen appreciation of the much we wish to give makes us feel peculiarly incompetent and we approach the task with eagerness tempered with humility.

It is our earnest desire to make as vivid as we can the spirit and ideals of Bukh, the man, without which no one can appreciate the deep desire to serve which permeates the original book. We have rearranged the material, amplifying some sections and curtailing and subordinating others, but have in no way changed the character of the book. We have based our changes on the results of our experience with the work in the Central School of Hygiene and *Physical* Education during the years 1923 to 1927, and on our achievements as shown by careful medical and physical examinations and tests.

I am indebted to my students at the Central School, and to my graduate teachers groups during the winters of 1924 to 1927, and to my class in 1926 to 1927 at Teachers College, Columbia University, and in the summer of 1925 at New York University, for their inspiration, help and criticism in class discussions. The opportunity of conducting these classes in theory and practice has greatly clarified my own conception and understanding of Fundamental Gymnastics.

To the first two American groups in Denmark, in the summers of 1926 and 1927, I wish to express my appreciation for their co-operation, keen study of and clear vision for the work.

To Dr. William Skarstrom,—his pupils who were **my**

first teachers, and his book "Gymnastic Teaching,"—
I owe whatever thorough, technical grasp of gymnastics
I may have.

Miss Vesterdal and I wish particularly to thank Miss
Flora Cutting for her earnest study resulting in a suc-
cessful adaptation for her students at the Wadleigh
High School, New York City.

It is our pleasure also to make appreciative mention
of those individuals in New York City who have made
valuable contributions in the application of Fundamental Gymnastics in the corrective and remedial field—
Mrs. Ella Biondi, New York Orthopedic Hospital; Miss
Miriam Sweeny; Miss Harriet Wilde; Miss Hazel
Kinzly, under the direction of Dr. Arthur Krida; and
of Miss Lillian Curtis Drew for her critical, technical
advice and suggestions.

We owe much to Dr. Stella S. Bradford, examining
physician at the Central School, for her interest, expert
diagnosis, and help in our study of the effects of Fundamental Gymnastics on our students; and to Miss
Helen Luffman and Miss May Fenner for their pains-
taking work upon the manuscript.

We extend our deepest gratitude to Miss Helen
McKinstry for her belief in us, for her unfailing encouragement, and for making this book possible through
her reviews and constructive criticism of the manuscript
in all stages of its preparation.

TABLE OF CONTENTS

1. Invented movements. 2. Non-definite type of
exercises. 3. Alternation of activity and rest.
4. Increased and unlimited range of movement.
5. Use of extremities as points of attachment and as
weight leverage. 6. Support of Stall Bar or helper
to increase the weight leverage. 7. Rhythmical continuity of movement. 8. Individual rhythms—
'Lack of Unison.' 9. No rigidity or tension. 10.
A strong self-testing element.

1. Terminology. 2. Use of starting positions. 3.
Movements. 4. Signals. 5. Admonitions and
stimulations. 6. Voice. 7. Different methods in
presenting work. 8. The lesson plan. 9. Marching.
10. Opening order.

1. Environmental factors. 2. Type and capacity of
a class: Adaptation for elementary grades; junior
and senior high schools; colleges and universities;
Y. M. C. A. and Y. W. C. A.; for special individuals;
normal schools of physical education. 3. General
principles in progression—within the lesson and from
lesson to lesson. 4. Speed. 5. Rhythm. 6. Specific principles in progression.

INTRODUCTORY CHAPTER

Within the past year a book has been published that makes no reference to *P*hysical Education but is nevertheless a most valuable addition to the library of every teacher who wishes to be called an educator in our particular field. *I* refer to "Modern Educational Theories" by *P*rofessor Boyd H. Bode.

We are accustomed to make extravagant claims for physical activities and have talked glibly of their health, educational, corrective, and recreative values.

When forced to become specific we have resorted to the trite statements that 'health is a by-product of muscular activity,' and 'physical activity becomes educational to the extent that it makes for a feeling of well being necessary to efficient mental growth and development.'

We cite the recreative values of games and sports to emphasize their character and citizenship training values, as though football and basketball were ordained to give birth to these abstract psychophysical attributes, irrespective of conditions and leadership.

In this respect *P*hysical Education has striven valiantly to keep pace with Liberal Education and its vague, high sounding objectives of harmonious development, social efficiency, self-realization and culture.

*P*rofessor Bode characterizes such objectives as having "the appearance of being a kind of New Year resolutions, formulated in conformity with the spirit of the occasion but with no thought of taking them seriously."[1]

In General Education, the violent reaction to such formulation of nebulous aims has resulted in the setting up of specific activities aimed at securing a list of specific abilities that "offers us something that is neither fish nor fowl." [2]

"If every specific activity means a corresponding specific ability, then the list, long as it is, is but a haphazard random sampling. Why not an ability to thread a needle, to sew on buttons, to climb a fence, and to be amiable toward one's mother-in-law? Why not, in short, reduce life as far as possible to the level of mechanical habit? On the other hand if there is such a thing as the training of general ability, what is the meaning of all the detail? Unless we have some sort of guiding philosophy in the determination of objectives, we get nowhere at all." [3]

"The notion . . . that our educational program must be guided by predetermined specific activities inevitably distracts our attention from general training. In so far as general training receives any recognition at all, it is left without any guiding principle." [4]

F. Bobbitt, the apostle of job analysis, contends that "Activity analysis is the beginning of all curriculum making. Find the activities which men perform, or those which they should perform: and train for those." [5]

Professor Bode replies that "Activity analysis does not determine objectives, but our objectives determine

[1] Bode, B. H., "Modern Educational Theories," pp. 73–74, by permission of The Macmillan Company, publishers.

[2] Ibid., p. 87.

[3] Ibid., p. 87.

[4] Ibid., p. 89.

[5] Bobbitt, F., "How to Make a Curriculum," p. 256, by permission of Houghton Mifflin Company, publishers.

what sort of facts are needed, and consequently how the method is to be used. In the end, as is only too apparent, activity analysis furnishes no objectives or ideals. It tells us what is but not what ought to be." [6]

"There is no escape from the everlasting paradox that a subject is more practical if we do not try too hard to make it practical. It is only by maintaining something of a disinterested or scientific attitude that we secure the margin of extra knowledge which enables us to meet emergencies. In the language of an advertisement announcing a blanket sale: 'It's the part that hangs over that keeps you warm.' " [7]

To quote *Professor Bode* still further, "We hear a great deal, for example, about 'child purposing' and about individual differences without a sufficiently counterbalancing emphasis upon the need of developing and directing the activities of pupils toward a preconceived end." [8]

" . . . the concept of democracy involves a program of living." [9]

"The life of the next generation will be different from ours, and it will be different in ways that we cannot foresee. How then can we prepare for it?"

"*Perhaps* the simplest answer to this question is that education should enable the individual to educate himself when the time comes." [10]

To the reader, interested only in acquiring new exercises, this lengthy preamble may seem another bit of pious admonishing far removed from consideration of the values and use of Fundamental Gymnastics. To

[6] Bode, B. H., "Modern Educational Theories," p. 112.
[7] Ibid., p. 296.
[8] Ibid., p. 33.
[9] Ibid., p. 346.
[10] Ibid., p. 238.

such, we sincerely hope this book will make no appeal. They belong to the age of "trainers" and "systems" and between them and the author and translators of this book there is nothing in common. The work of Niels Bukh is a repudiation of systems, formalities, and artificialities. It is equally far removed, in its concepts, from the specific objectives of "education for farming and farmers."

As taught in Ollerup, Denmark, the work is applied to meet the needs of boys and girls, the majority of whom have had a part in making, to quote Ex-Governor Lowden, "the most highly developed agricultural life the world has ever known." They return, from the Peoples Colleges, to their model farms to continue the development of their lives and their work with a broader conception of life and its interests and activities. Their adult education makes for a broadening, not a restriction, of their horizons, and America could profit much by a study of Denmark's objectives and ideals.

The work of Niels Bukh is internationally recognized as a valuable contribution to 'programs of living.' As Miss Andrews mentions, his book has been translated into nine different languages and seventy thousand copies have been sold in Germany alone. We can talk of world-fellowship and a League of Nations, but, as Professor Bode comments, "It has sometimes been pointed out by critics abroad that we Americans tend to regard our institutions and practices as final; that our minds are closed, so that we are less tolerant and less progressive than other countries. No more serious criticism could be made than this. In so far as it is true we are not democratic, whatever we may choose to call ourselves." [11]

[11] Bode, B. H., "Modern Educational Theories," p. 236.

And again, "We have been afraid to tolerate other religions and other races and have organized against them. We have set up standards of patriotism which made it an act of disloyalty to think." [12]

In 1923, when Niels Bukh came to America with a group of students, the reaction against formalized activities of any type was at its height. We had ceased to defend "systems," but the camp of the formalists and the reactionaries were still prepared for battle. We talked in terms of general and specific objectives and abilities, and the advocates of each group saw little of value in the ideas and practices of the other.

We talked theoretically in terms of the millennium, while there were as yet inadequate facilities and leadership for even the most out-grown of our practices.

Niels Bukh demonstrated little that was new in exercises, but changed old emphases. He exhibited a method of formalizing general and specific developmental activities with all the old tension and rigidity made conspicuously absent. The possibilities in the use of such a flow of activity—vigorous, stimulating, free and satisfying to the performer,—were apparent to the great majority of the teachers in his audiences.

That something we call Fate, which seems to function quite independently of our conscious choice or effort, placed Karen Vesterdal, one of Mr. Bukh's group, in the Central School of Hygiene and Physical Education for the year 1923–24. This intimate contact with Mr. Bukh's work, its underlying principles and its results, stimulated Miss Andrews to continue her investigation of its values through a summer spent at the Peoples College in Ollerup. She returned, enthusiastic and eager to make a test of the work, with adaptations, in the

12 Bode, B. H., "Modern Educational Theories," p. 287.

Central School. With reluctance, it must be confessed, she was permitted to give this work exclusively to one class for one semester. Long before this experimental period came to an end, the enthusiasm of students and their joy in the work was so manifest, it was not surprising to find our mid-term physical and medical examinations proved conclusively that the results had justified the means. Since that time, the gymnastic work in the Central School has more and more been adapted in conformity with Mr. Bukh's methods and emphases, while, at the same time, Miss Andrews has built these methods and activities upon the scholarly and scientifically sound principles elucidated by William Skarstrom in his "Gymnastic Teaching." The criticism that the Central School is teaching formalized activities exclusively can be met in no better way than by mentioning the amount of time given to such work. The three years of the course include a total of 810 hours of practical work. Of these, 440 are devoted to games and sports, 165 to dancing, and 195 to class and individual gymnastics. Of the 205 hours given to special method courses, gymnastics lay claim to but 30, with sports and games occupying 130.

Our acknowledged interest in Mr. Bukh's work brought a constantly increasing number of requests from teachers throughout the U. S. A. for information and opportunity to study it. When we failed in our endeavor to bring Mr. Bukh to America, for either a summer or a winter course, he suggested, as an alternative, that the Central School, acting as his representative, select from among the applicants those women instructors in physical education who were really interested in the theoretical and educational values of his methods and activities, and take them to Denmark for a six weeks' summer course. With his ever keen appreciation of the dangers attendant on the too rapid and thoughtless absorption of anything new, and the possible inability of many teachers to study work in Denmark and still keep eyes and thoughts on American needs and standards, his suggestion of the summer course carried with it the absolute requirement that Miss Andrews go with the group and interpret the theory and the activities in terms of American conditions and ideals.

Two such summer courses in Denmark have borne astonishing fruit in the sane and critical but appreciative interest developed in the work by the fifty-four women who have lived for six weeks in the Ollerup environment of culture, beauty, and charm, and in daily contact with Niels Bukh,—the patriot, the educator, and the man of ideals, vision, courage, and honor.

As an outgrowth of the very general interest in Fundamental Gymnastics and of the desire, both of those Americans who go to Denmark and those who cannot, to have a clean cut exposition of his principles and methods, Mr. Bukh has designated Miss Andrews, as "that one of my students who most clearly analyzes my work and thoroughly understands my aims," to prepare an adaptation, and revision of the English translation for American use.

The book has not been revised with the paramount purpose of presenting Fundamental Gymnastics as a new fad, a substitute for what we already have, or as a solution of our problems in physical education—no, not even to solve those of our formalized activities. The purpose of physical education in a democracy is to do its part in education's task of building a program of living. The exponents of Fundamental Gymnastics endorse these activities and methods as valuable tools for use in the building of the foundations of organic development, neuro-muscular control and bodily freedom, upon which the superstructure of activities, skills and interests for efficient living and for leisure may be erected.

Fundamental Gymnastics is neither a 'hard work' nor a 'high grade play' subject, but vigorous, stimulating, basically developmental and bodily conditioning activities. The keen satisfaction of the performer is expressive of the effectiveness of the work and thereby enhances it.

Systems of physical education have passed into the discard along with "the safe and elegant imbecility of classical learning" but the time has not come for abandoning the attempt at a 'logical organization' of our physical activities, dependent in large measure upon a psychological organization that will satisfy the desires of childhood and adult life and, of even greater importance, adequately provide for their growth and developmental needs.

Education for specific skills, abilities and attributes for vocation and recreation is one of our American ideals, and one to be fostered at all hazards.

When the day comes,—and we pray it may come speedily,—that our children and youth are provided with those minimum essentials for normal growth and development that necessitate adequate space, outdoor facilities, time allotment and constructive leadership, it will then be time to relinquish our formalized activities. Until such time, it is our contention that Fundamental Gymnastics will be found to be a most valuable and interesting substitute for much of the formalized and restricted material in current use. With such a point of view it is believed the intelligent and thoughtful reader will be in perfect sympathy, and that this book will do much to limit the use of its practical material to those teachers who, with justifiable conservatism, demand a sound theoretical background for all new work.

HELEN McKINSTRY

FUNDAMENTAL GYMNASTICS

CHAPTER I

Values and Objectives of Fundamental Gymnastics in Terms of American Ideals and Conditions

The type of formalized activity, designated as Fundamental Gymnastics, has the value, common to all gymnastics, of being adaptable to use whenever and wherever conditions of time, space and equipment make artificial exercises necessary.

The unique values lie, not in new forms of activity, but in the range of the movements and in the methods of teaching which give a more stimulating and organically developmental quality to the activity, and result in a personal satisfaction in accomplishment that is not emphasized in gymnastics more formally taught with range of movements definitely limited.

Fundamental Gymnastics are in no sense to be considered as 'fundamental activities' for children, but they are basically developmental, organically stimulating, corrective and enjoyable artificial exercises, given for the purpose of reaching specific objectives in general development and control, or as a preparation for the acquisition and pursuance of activities that are intrinsically valuable and satisfying. It cannot be too strongly stated that Fundamental Gymnastic exercises are never objectives or ends in themselves, but their place in the physical education program is that of emergency tools.

There is no question that the ideal program of 'big muscle activities' for children should be, in so far as possible, a natural one based on child needs and capacities. Where ideal conditions exist and a child can spend the needed three to five hours a day in play, out of doors or in an adequate play room, there should be no need for formalized activities. It is a truism to state that such ideal provisions are not yet universal in America, and that the physical education program in elementary and high schools must, for some time to come, contain formal elements. Where such need exists, it is our contention that the less formally taught exercises of Fundamental Gymnastics provide a better substitute for natural activities than do the more military and exact and less interesting exercises which are still in use in many schools. The inadequate physical education program of the past has not given to the average adult of today the organic and neuro-muscular development necessary for efficient living. Coupled with this, the economic pressure and present-day lack of time, space and leadership in wholesome adult recreation, bear abundant fruit in the constantly increasing number of nervous disorders. Our adult population has a poor physical foundation and is living too hard and fast for its limited physical capital. For adults, then, there must be provided a *get fit* and *keep fit* program of activities that, with the limited facilities provided, can be given to large groups and be led by one teacher. Activities must be taught in one or two lessons a week that can be used by individuals in their daily, ten to fifteen minute, *keep fit* allotment of time at home and in the ordinary cramped space of the modern room. To meet such a need, Fundamental Gymnastics provide a stimulating and interesting type of activity that can be suited to individual needs.

In speaking of adult needs, Mr. Bukh states his aim for Fundamental Gymnastics to be a "thorough working and toning up of the whole body." In two picturesque metaphors he stresses the importance and necessity of using more than natural methods in the counteraction of unfavorable conditions. "The hard-pan of the moorlands must be broken and the tough roots of the heather removed before the soil can be made to yield. A field, the fertility of which is impaired by bad cultivation and mismanagement, first needs thorough working and a new supply of substances which make it fertile before it will again yield good crops. Likewise, the clay of which the artist makes his models must first be thoroughly softened and worked before it can be shaped by skillful hands to express in its lines the beauty of form and character that is the master's ideal."

If the body is to be the ready and efficient vehicle of expression it must be free, supple, strong and perfectly under control. The limited amount and variety of physical activity in modern life has made this ideal impossible, and the deficiencies in these bodily attributes is seen in the stiffness, weakness and awkwardness of the body at rest and in motion.

There are three main headings under which faults and lacks in development can be classified,—(1) stiffness, obvious in movements in the joints, spine and muscles; (2) lack of power, shown in the use of the muscles; and (3) awkwardness or lack of freedom and co-ordination evidenced in the movements of the body.

If these faults are to be corrected and the deficiencies met, the objectives to be set up are *flexibility, strength* and *co-ordination* or *agility*. Flexibility must take the place of stiffness, ligamentous tension must be released, and over-contracted muscles normalized before a perfect relation between the different segments of the body can be achieved and an adequate musculature built.

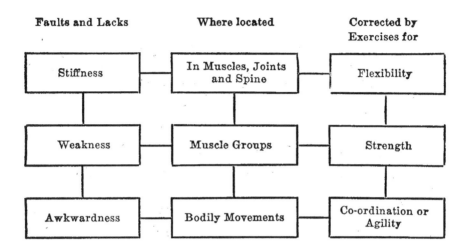

Faults and Lacks	Where located	Corrected by Exercises for
Stiffness	In Muscles, Joints and Spine	Flexibility
Weakness	Muscle Groups	Strength
Awkwardness	Bodily Movements	Co-ordination or Agility

The body must be so efficient that it can meet more than an aesthetic demand. Good posture is unfortunately too often stressed as the first and final objective of gymnastics. The body must be able to respond immediately and with accuracy in any situation calling for spontaneous action, and do this with the greatest efficiency and the least expenditure of effort. The poise of the body at rest, and the carriage and efficient use of the body in action, should be the criteria for judging how thoroughly fundamental work has been done. In summary, fundamental gymnastic activities are:

1. *Corrective*

> Good habits are substituted for poor ones. Exaggerated curves of the spine are normalized. Stiffness in the joints is overcome and a free range of movement is made possible. Muscle groups are strengthened.

2. *Developmental*

> The vigorous and rhythmic nature of the ac-
> tivity results in marked organic stimulation,
> affecting the circulatory, respiratory, digestive,
> excretory and heat regulating mechanisms of the
> body.

3. *Co-ordinative*

> Neuro-muscular skill—co-ordination, agility,
> rhythm, freedom and grace of movement—is in-
> creased.

The standard of bodily perfection differs little in civi-
lized countries, nor has the ideal of physical beauty
been greatly changed by time or race. It is true, however, that the particular conception of health and fitness
varies somewhat in different countries dependent upon
and coalescent with the prevailing utility ideal. There
is, therefore, a practical basis for the statement that a
"system" cannot be transplanted, in toto, from one country to another, and that a type of work which adequately
meets the needs of one nation has not been proven to
be of universal value by virtue of its worth to one group.
What others have found valuable in their experience
bears evidence of some worth for us, and if we, in
America, can subscribe to a common utility need, if
an activity can be adapted to our own situation, and if
we test our results carefully, there need be no hesitation
in accepting and using a type of work that has been
planned for another country. Our purpose must be to
provide the means and the method for correcting and
perfecting bodily conditions, and one great task is the
selection of those types of activity that can best meet
the needs of individuals. If we are to secure results,

our aim must be accurate, our tools carefully selected, and the ultimate objective clearly before us. In the words of Niels Bukh: "As the farmer has the harvest in his thoughts when he cultivates the earth in the spring, so the leader should have the vision of his ideal standard of development always before him as the best guide in his work."

CHAPTER II

OUTSTANDING CHARACTERISTICS

Before undertaking the discussion of the special characteristics of Fundamental Gymnastics, it is important to explain the present confusion of terms by which the work has become known.

The two names most commonly in use today are 'Danish' and 'Fundamental.' No one has the desire to be pedantic and force upon this type of activity a name that does not apply, and possibly it would be wise not to qualify it by any distinguishing term. However, since this book is a translation as well as a revision and adaptation, it is not advisable to take such a stand at present.

Since 'Fundamental' is the translation of the Danish terms *Primitiv* and *Grund,* Mr. Bukh advocates its use as being most descriptive of his work. The fifty-four American teachers of physical education (representing training in seventeen Normal Schools of Physical Education) who have studied with Mr. Bukh in Denmark, also favor this name as being the most significant one to use.

Fundamental Gymnastics must not in any sense be interpreted *fundamental activities,* nor should it be implied that this work precedes or takes the place of a natural activity program. Since its emphasis is on the correction of faults and the development of strength, it

9

may well be termed basic, preparatory work and should be used as such in a program of physical education. When gymnastics are included in a program it is advisable that this type should be given before all other types of gymnastics i.e., non-definite before defiinite work.

The term 'Danish' applied to this work is in every sense a misnomer since it may apply to any one of the several kinds of work now being taught in Danish schools. Also 'Danish' at once links it with other great systems of gymnastics which have swept this country in the past. It immediately takes on the appearance of that which it is not—a system.

Mr. Bukh strongly objects to having his work labeled a "system," appreciating how readily many fall into a rut and teach a *system* rather than *people*. We are through with systems in America. They have had their day. We must think of people and their needs and develop a *type of work* based upon such needs. It will be necessary to add to and change it in many particulars to meet the needs and capacities of the individuals being taught. Mr. Bukh is continually testing his work, changing and developing it, as his experience broadens.

OUTSTANDING CHARACTERISTICS OF FUNDAMENTAL GYMNASTICS

1. *Invented Movements—Formalized Activities*

Mr. Bukh has made an attempt to take useful movements of free athletics and use them (artificially) to develop power and freedom which, once gained, can be turned to recreative ends. The athlete's need of powerful and agile legs may be acquired without the use of track, hurdles or jumping standards. These exercises are not to be given as mimetic activities nor as a substitute for play. They should be classified as invented movements under the main heading of formalized activities, and they may be taught either formally or informally.

2. *Non-definite Type of Exercises*

The great majority of exercises in Fundamental Gymnastics can be classified as *non-definite* movements, as compared with *definite* gymnastics which emphasize sustained positions. Both types are described at length by Dr. William Skarstrom in his book on "Gymnastic Teaching," pages 75–78. The following is an excerpt from his discussion on non-definite exercises.

"Exercises of the non-definite type are relatively complex, widely distributed movements, not readily capable of sharp definition or standardization; their various elements are so blended and interdependent that the exercises cannot easily or to any great extent be divided into component parts without destroying or at least changing their character. They are usually continuous i.e., the movements are repeated in smooth or at any rate immediate alternation and sequence, not separated by sustained positions. The momentum or recoil of one movement gives the impetus for the next. . . ."

He goes on to say that because of the vigorous nature of these exercises they are "effective in stimulating the circulatory, respiratory, digestive and excretory organs as well as all parts of the heat regulating mechanism . . ." and "the fact that such exercises usually are done with rhythmic continuity emphasizes their general organic effects."

3. *Alternation of Activity and Rest*

Activity alternating with rest is a feature of each exercise, and characteristic of the change from exercise to exercise.

An inflexible student has a very limited range of movement. It is important for a beginner, at least, to be conscious of his possible range in each movement, passing from the limit of action to the most complete relaxation in the recoil.

Utilizing the momentum adds to the force and effectiveness of the exercise and, through increasing the range, quickly brings about a flexible condition.

The entire lesson is built upon this principle of exertion and relaxation. By continually shifting action from one part of the body to another,—without entire cessation of activity,—tired muscles are given a rest period and work can be prolonged, to an increasing degree, without fatigue. Lessons composed of 35–50 exercises then become possible. Spectators, who do not take this principle of "rest-in-motion" into consideration, judge the work as "too strenuous" and the lesson appears to them more like torture than fun.

4. *Increased and Unlimited Range of Movement*

Fundamental Gymnastics are not given to develop extreme strength or produce that exaggerated suppleness which is necessary for acrobatic skill. Their only purpose is to approximate the ideal and natural condition which has been lost as a result of a limited amount and degree of activity.

In stretching the hamstring muscles, they are not the only group affected since the lower back is also straightened. Hamstring muscles are the first to tighten after a period of rest, and as the demands of daily life require little activity, the knees are flexed more than half the time. Therefore, in a gymnastic lesson, to correct this condition by conscious and forceful stretching will not, to any great extent, overcorrect or produce a loose jointed condition or hyper-extension in this region. Much work in knee bending is also given for the opposite effect—that of strengthening the legs. The condition of hyper-extended knees is usually associated with a tipped pelvis and hollow back. Correcting the angle of the pelvis by straightening the hollow back, and getting the weight distribution properly adjusted, usually eliminates this appearance of hyper-extended knees. It has been proven by tests that supple students have taken all the flexibility work required without increasing their suppleness in this region.

In Fundamental Gymnastics the individual is not limited by being urged to reach and hold exact positions. In bendings, twistings, flingings, the bodily movements are limited only by joint and muscle restrictions. This is far easier for a beginner than the attainment of exact positions, but later on, in advanced work, the range of movement may be made smaller and the "kinesthetic sense" necessary in quick, accurate motor responses be developed.

5. *Use of Extremities as Points of Attachment and as Weight Leverage*

To localize and increase the force of some movements, unique starting positions are used e.g., hands grasp the ankles, knees or feet. In some movements the weight of arms, legs or trunk is the agent employed to increase the force and range through producing greater leverage.

See Chapter III (2) Use of Starting Positions. (3) Movements.

6. *Support of Stall Bar or Helper to Increase the Weight Leverage*

Many exercises are done at the stall bars or with a helper. In stall-bar work where arms or legs or both are fixed, the starting position is stabilized, thereby making possible an increase in the force and range of movements, as well as their localization in a desired region. In work with partners where legs are locked, or hands clasped, or bodies braced, work is made stronger and more effective and, at the same time, intensely interesting. In couple work, either at the stall bars or on the floor, it is advisable that partners be of approximately the same size and strength.

7. *Rhythmical Continuity of Movement*

Continuity of movement is characteristic of a lesson in Fundamental Gymnastics. The unique manner of "going" from one exercise to another gives the class the feeling of progress through continuous action. This is true even in beginners' classes where the change from exercise to exercise is ragged and incomplete. In advanced classes the changes are almost perfect. Since the positions of "at ease" and "attention" are conspicuous by their absence, this transition from one exercise to another in time becomes so smooth and rhythmical that the work often falsely suggests a learned drill.

8. *Individual Rhythms—"Lack of Unison"*

Exercises are individualized to the extent that the movements of the more flexible students in a class are in no way restricted or inhibited to give the appearance of class unison. Class work will lack the uniformity, precision and perfection of movement that pleases the eye until such time as the least flexible, weakest and most unco-ordinated student has developed average or superior ability.

9. *No Rigidity or Tension*

"Extension without tension" is characteristic of the work. Exercises should be done in a free manner with few held positions. Where these do occur, in response movements, there must be no tenseness or strain in the execution. Free breathing is urged in all work and is especially to be emphasized in some of the strength exercises where the chest muscles are liable to be fixated during the performance of a strong trunk stretching or chest lifting.

10. *A Strong Self-Testing Element*

These exercises cannot be classified as *stunts* but many of them have a strong inherent self-testing element and because of this are *fun* to do. By voluntary practice outside of class, many students perfect exercises of this 'trick' or 'stumping' type, and get keen satisfaction in accomplishment as they exhibit their newly acquired skill at the next lesson hour.

In summary, Fundamental Gymnastics are characterized by a stream of activity without rigidity, tension or inhibition, a stretching, strengthening, co-ordinating of the body in all its parts with an accompanying exhilaration and sense of satisfaction, increased endurance and achievement. As we successfully adapt this work to our own teaching situations it becomes, not merely a foreign importation—a fad—but a most serviceable tool that will meet a definite need in our physical education program in America.

CHAPTER III

TEACHING TECHNIQUE

1. *Terminology*

The nomenclature used throughout this book is based, in general, on that found in "Gymnastic Teaching" by William Skarstrom, published by the American Physical Education Association. Although there is no standard nomenclature in use in America, Dr. Skarstrom's terminology is the most generally used in schools of Physical Education. Therefore, with a few changes, it has been used here as a criterion for many starting positions and movements.

In some cases there has been a return to the older Swedish terms because of their conciseness or clarity. In instances where long descriptions have been used by Dr. Skarstrom to designate certain positions, liberty has been taken in shortening these to conform to the general character of the work. Much of the nomenclature in use today, in Denmark as well as America, owes its origin to the Swedish terminology, and hence a great similarity has been found to exist. For example, in the starting position *wing standing,* Chapter V, No. I, the term *hip standing* is given as an alternative. There has been some question of the advisability of returning to the use of *wing standing,* but it has been preferred by many teachers as more adequately descriptive of the position. *Hip grasp standing,* frequently used, is taken with the hands resting on the hip bones, wrists straight,

16

thumbs back and fingers pointing forward. In Mr. Bukh's *wing standing* the hands are placed much lower, almost on the hip joints, and the wrists are relaxed. In the former position, *hip grasp,* there is a tendency to hunch the shoulders with a definite feeling of tenseness in keeping the wrists straight. This is entirely overcome in the lower position of *wing standing.*

2. *Use of Starting Positions*

A position from which a movement is started and to which the movement returns at the completion of the exercise is called a *starting position.* In Fundamental Gymnastics the return to the initial starting position is frequently omitted by the blending of two exercises, in which case the class is not carried back to the starting position of the first exercise but into the starting position of the succeeding exercise.

Progression in the use of starting positions, involving the lower extremities, is usually secured by decreasing the width of the base of support e.g., *stride standing* to the narrower base in *walk standing* or to the *erect standing* position.

The raising of the center of gravity, through a change in arm positions, has been another factor employed in making exercises more difficult e.g., an exercise performed with the hands resting on the hips is made progressively more difficult by raising the hands to *bend, arm side,* and *stretch* positions. Thus, exercises taken from increasingly difficult starting positions of the legs (through narrowing the base), combined with a raising of the center of gravity (by changing the positions of the arms), trains the student in weight distribution, and calls for a higher degree of balance and greater control of the body in action.

Mr. Bukh uses starting positions, not only for the purposes just described, but as important parts of the exercises themselves. They are not mere factors in progression nor are they chosen from the point of view of "dressing up" an exercise, but are selected primarily for their great utility value to the exercises. Since this is his object, a starting position can be changed very little without greatly changing the character of the exercise.

A starting position may definitely limit the range of a movement but by so doing localize it, as in *hand knee standing trunk twisting with arm flinging*. The starting position may increase the force of the movement, as in *half grasp stride bow standing trunk springing*. In this the hand grasps the ankle to give greater leverage, localize the movement, and increase its force. When the particular need for such a starting position is no longer evident, the starting position for the same exercise may be varied e.g., *stride bow standing trunk springing* with the arms hanging free. In naming a starting position, the customary order is, arms, legs, trunk, e.g., *neck stride bow standing*.

3. *Movements*

A movement is the act of passing from one position to another. There are a great many *blended compound* or *composite* exercises in Fundamental Gymnastics, which can not easily be broken up or divided without changing the character of the exercises. As one part of an exercise blends into the next part there is no definite demarcation between them.

SPECIAL FEATURES OF MOVEMENTS AND THEIR USE

In Fundamental Gymnastics the movements are free and of wide range. The force of a movement and its range are both increased by increasing leverage e.g., (1) *half wing stride standing trunk twisting with arm flinging* (ex. no. 53); (2) *stride standing arm flinging between cross and fly* (ex. no. 30); in these two examples the arms are the levers increasing the range of the movement; (3) *jump between squat sitting and stride standing* (ex. no. 7); (4) *neck stride angle standing trunk springing* (ex. no. 22). In (3) and (4) the weight of the body is the increasing force.

With a beginning class, the shortened muscles and ligamentous tension of the majority of the students, permit of a very limited range of movement. As the work progresses, the increase in range and freedom of movement is very marked.

The vigor with which a movement is taken may, with a less flexible member of the class, result in a hollowing of the lower back and a thrusting of the head forward. This is due to lack of freedom in the shoulder girdle.

This is not an important objection, since much work is given to definitely straighten the neck and lower back, and also because the condition will soon be remedied through the stretching of shortened muscles. The teacher's admonitions should call frequent attention to the defects in execution, and there must be conscious effort toward correction on the part of the pupil. Where it seems advisable, students may work in pairs, one (as helper) kneeling by the performer and controlling the action by placing his hands on the performer's abdomen and lower back, thus decreasing the mobility of this region.

The emphasis in Fundamental Gymnastics is not placed on posture (as a static condition), to the degree that the normal, free action of the spine in all directions is limited. In securing a free and poised carriage, suppleness, freedom and muscular sufficiency of the spine are considered fundamental to the acquisition of neuro-muscular control. As soon as the chest and shoulder girdle are freed and the head does not project forward on the execution of exercises, definite work for strengthening the neck and back is begun.

The exercises in Fundamental Gymnastics, when carefully chosen and skillfully taught, have the effect on the body of a moulding process and bring about a normal relationship between different parts and segments, resulting in poise and control at rest and in action.

4. Signals

In any formalized group activity, such as gymnastics, there must be a definite method of presenting work. The teacher names and describes the position to be taken or the movement to be done, and designates a certain time when this is to be acted upon in unison by the class. This is called the *signal,* and it is composed of three parts.

Preparatory part: this is a clear and vigorous explanation of what is to be done—the description of the exercise or the name of the movement—and may be given while the class is still performing the last exercise.

Pause: the second part of the signal is the pause during which the student "thinks" about the new exercise. The teacher decides at what moment the executive word must be given in order to achieve a natural and satisfactory change of movement.

The executive word: this is the final signal and must be spoken in a pleasant but clear and concise manner, to be instantly understood by all.

The executive word for response movements may be given in the imperative form of the verb, such as "bend!" "fling!", "lift!", "stretch!", which names specifically the action for the movement; examples—"Chest—lift!" —"relax!" "Knees—stretch!"—"bend!" A numerical executive signal may also be given in a response movement, by using the present participle of the verb in the preparatory signal, and numbers for the final signal,— "Chest lifting—one!"—"two!" To avoid monotony, if repetition of the same response movement is desired, it is a good plan to use both imperative and numerical signals, one following the other.

In most starting positions, simple or compound, the final signal is in the imperative. "Hands on hips— place!", "Hands on hips and feet sideways—place!" Where three regions of the body are included, as in *neck stride bow standing,* two signals may be given e.g., "Hands on neck and feet sideways—place!" After this movement has been executed the next signal may be "Trunk downward—bend!" This is a rather long and involved process and necessary only for beginners. It is possible to have a class, very early in their course of lessons, respond accurately to the above movement by the following signal, "Placing the left foot sideways, hands on neck, trunk downward—bend!"

If it is desired to have the class go, without a pause, from one movement to a starting position which involves a change in the position of the feet, e.g., to go from a *stride standing position* to a *hand squat sitting position,* the following type of signal could be used,— "Bringing the left foot to the right, hands on floor— knees deep—bend!" This signal must be given as the preceding movement, from a stride position, is being executed.

SUGGESTIONS FOR SIGNALS FOR MOVEMENTS

When it is desirable to go from one exercise into the next exercise without a stop, it is possible to time the executive word so that the change may be a rhythmical one and without breaking the continuity of the movement. While one movement is being executed, the teacher gives the preparatory part of the next exercise in such a manner as to include the starting position as well as the movement. After a short pause the final signal is given. This method will not make for uniformity of movement at first. A few students will respond quickly and accurately and the others will get into the movement as promptly as they can, but, after a few lessons, the class as a whole will enjoy the fun of reaching the next exercise on time. This gives a "game-like" element to the work. With advanced classes, these changes will become rhythmical and there will be complete unison of movement.

TIMING OF SIGNALS

In most instances, when going from exercise to exercise, or from an exercise to the next starting position, a final signal may be given when the arms are moving away from the body e.g., the class is executing—*stride standing arm flinging between* $\times$ *and fly* and the exercise to follow it is—*neck stride bow standing trunk springing.* The signal, *"Hands on neck trunk downward —bend!"*, is given just as the arms are moving upward from the $\times$ to *fly* position. From the *fly* position the hands are then placed on the neck and the trunk bent downward. The next signal is then "Trunk springing— begin!"

It is advisable to keep movements as simple as possible so that the description may be short and give a vivid mental picture. If an exercise involves two regions of the body (arms and legs) it is better to start the legs and then give the signal for the arms while the leg movement is being executed.

It is difficult to give these signals at first but very soon, and with a little practice, it becomes simple.

When a starting position is included in the preparatory signal, the use of technical terms should be avoided. Instead of saying "Half wing stride standing—trunk twisting with arm flinging—begin!" say *"P*lacing right hand on the hip and left foot sideways—trunk twisting with arm flinging—begin!" or in the exercise—*back clasp knee bow sitting* (when the class is already in kneeling position) the signal may be "Clasping hands behind the back—on heels—sit!"

SIGNALS FOR RHYTHMICAL WORK

In starting rhythmical movements the final signal is usually, "begin!" "go!" or "now!" The cessation of a movement must receive important consideration. The *stopping* signal should be given with just as much tone and clarity as the *starting* signal if the attention and interest is to be held for the next exercise. Too often "stop!" is drawled out in a lackadaisical manner, and the class, engaged in performing an exercise, responds to this "let down" in the teacher's voice by diminished vigor in work.

Signals are necessary in a gymnastic lesson but they are not the most important part of the instruction. In cases where the signal plays too large a part, it is a relic of the old military system accepted without further thought or understanding. A friendly relationship must exist between the class and teacher—a reciprocal interest and good will—and the signals and the whole instruction must bear evidence of this.

5. *Admonitions and Stimulations*

Guidance in the performance of the exercise, correction of movements or positions, and encouragement to try again, are just as important factors in teaching as is the signal, and all are included in what is called *instruction*. If the teacher is thoroughly interested and alive to the need of *teaching individuals rather than exercises,* admonitions and cues will become a natural part of his instruction.

6. *Voice*

The teacher's voice is a tremendous power for good work. Through his voice a teacher makes his work live. In his voice he has the power to denote the type of movement which is desired—slow—quick—strong. In other words, the voice must be expressive of the movement to be done, never monotonous, never impatient, always clear, friendly and encouraging.

7. *Different Methods in Presenting Work*

Everything that is said and done by the teacher before an exercise is started is part of the presentation of the exercise. Such presentation must leave no question in the minds of the students as to what is required of them. Several methods may be emloyed:

(a) *Imitation*

The imitation method may be used successfully in non-definite or rhythmical work. The teacher executes a movement and the class follows her as accurately as possible. It is valuable in presenting new work as well as in some co-ordination exercises.

(b) *Description*

An exercise is clearly and concisely described. This is used to good advantage in familiar work, and where exercises are comparatively simple and easy to execute. It is also useful in rhythmical work where continuity of movement from exercise to exercise is desired.

(c) *Combination of Imitation and Description*

The combination of description and imitation may be used in presenting new and rather difficult or long exercises. In this method important points of the exercise may be emphasized, and the visual as well as auditory impression will be very helpful to the class.

8. *The Lesson Plan*

The lesson plan in Fundamental Gymnastics is similar to that for the more definite type of work, in that exercises for all parts of the body,—arms, legs, neck, back, abdomen, and side or lateral movements are used. In Fundamental Gymnastics, however, exercises must include *flexibility, strength, and agility* producing types of work, as well as an alternating use of trunk and extremities. Thus, in the lesson, it is essential to consider *regions* worked, and also the *effect* of the work upon such regions. The new teacher, when preparing his lessons, should note both effect and grouping of the various exercises, that he may be sure to include an equal distribution of flexibility, strength and agility work, and also a suitable versatility, alternation and progression. A skeletal lesson plan will be found in the appendix, page 174. This outline does not represent a fixed plan but merely a guide and example to be followed in the construction of lessons.

DIVISIONS OF THE LESSON

The lesson may be divided into three main divisions.

A. 1. Warming up—general, light, introductory work—all muscles brought into action to produce the desired hygienic and physiological effects.

    2. More localized work; including *bendings, twistings* and *over extensions* of the spine (especially in the dorsal and cervical regions), stretching of hamstring and pectoral muscles, strengthening of back and abdominal muscles, and the extensors and flexors of arms and legs.

Co-ordination exercises such as low hops and jumps, swingings, bendings, and stretchings of arms and legs are interposed between the more vigorous trunk exercises.

B.   Then follows the stronger work;—in pairs,

either on the floor or at the stall bars. The use of an individual or bar, as a point of attachment, gives a better support, and increases the strength of the work. It is now advisable to decrease the vigor of the lesson by introducing marching steps, easy running, or song games—that stress freedom and poise in movement.

C. The third division of the lesson may or may not be added. This part consists of agility exercises on the floor and apparatus.

The subdivisions a, b, c, d, e, etc. (see sample lesson plan in appendix, page 174) and also (Chapter IX. B—Combinations), are made with the idea of helping the teacher remember the sequence of exercises in a long table. Each of these subdivisions should include work for different parts of the body, but the exercises should be taken from the same or nearly allied starting positions. The exercises should follow each other in such a way that an easy and natural change is made to the next starting position, exercise, or group of exercises. Thus the whole table will hang together, and the sequence of exercises flow on without interruption.

It will be noted that *balance* and *breathing* exercises, as special groups, are omitted. At first, *movement* is stressed rather than *position*. In the early lessons there is ample opportunity to test weight distribution by the use of an easy balance movement. In advanced work, as the range of a movement is decreased, a balance movement becomes a balance position calling for a high degree of muscle sense and co-ordination. Breathing is naturally induced throughout the lesson by the vigorous rhythmical nature of the work. It is important that

normal breathing be emphasized in each exercise, so
that no tenseness or constriction occurs.

9. *Marching*

Mr. Bukh uses marching and running almost entirely
for gaining freedom of carriage, and for the purpose of
getting a class into the gymnasium and advantageously
arranged for gymnastic instruction. Emphasis is placed
on an easy, free carriage while the body is in motion,
and on a step that resembles the natural walk. In Denmark, classes sing as they walk around the room. Where
this has been tried in America, it has been found effective in creating a pleasant atmosphere.

Alignment: Files of 2 or 3, depending on the size of
the class, "line up" behind appointed
leaders.

Signal: (after the appointed leaders)
"Two and two forward—go!"

Numbering: As the class walks around the room the
"counting off" may be done in rhythm
with the steps. The accompanying diagram
indicates the order of numbering when
the class is in double file.

2 4 1 3 5 2 4 1 3 5 2 4 1 3 5

← 1 3 5 2 4 1 3 5 2 4 1 3 5 2 4 ←

Signal: "By two's (three's, four's, or
five's)—count off!"

American teachers of *Physical Education* are so familiar with marching tactics that only the following somewhat different steps are described here.

(a) *Free Walk*

> Emphasis is laid upon a free natural step with no exaggerated military stiffness or tension. The body weight is carried forward over the advancing foot, "heel, ball and toe" striking the floor almost simultaneously. The light step forward is followed by a strong "push off" with the rear foot, ankle well extended, as the weight is transferred. The arms hang straight and swing freely from the shoulders with an easy forward and backward motion. The chest is held high and over the forward foot. The walking of a well-trained class should sound as though they were treading on a carpeted floor.
>
> Signal: "Free walk—go!"

Faults and Corrective Admonitions or Cues

Too long a stride: "Shorter steps"
Weight back: "Weight forward"
Little or no ankle action: "Use your ankles"
Heavy step: "Lighter step"
No push off from rear foot: "Push off from rear foot"
Chest low: "Chest high"
Shoulders high and stiff: "Shoulders free and low"
Head forward: "Push up with the back of the head"

Arms bent and swung across body: "Arms swing straight and from the shoulders"

Hips not held firm: "Contract hip muscles"

Leg action not from the hip joint: "Free stride"

(b) *Firm Walk*

This is a slow, steady and exaggerated step and is nothing more than a knee lifting combined with walking. The value of the exercise lies in the stretching and freeing of hip and knee joints. The arms, in opposition to the leg movement, swing freely forward and backward to the height of the shoulders. The position of the head and chest is the same as in "free walk." The movements may be gradually decreased in range until a natural walk is again resumed. This walk helps in counteracting bad habits of posture and freeing cramped and ungainly movements.

(See illustration, page 161.)

Signal: "Firm walk—go!"

(c) *Kick Walk*

There is a strong extension in all joints as each leg is alternately kicked forward.

Signal: "With kicking step—forward—go!"

Marching or running with turns, and change steps, leg swinging and side steps, are often inserted as a "relief" activity between the more strenuous groups of exercises. Emphasis upon proper carriage of the body is always stressed.

10. *Opening Order*

In order that a gymnastic lesson may be started and conducted in a quick and efficient manner, the spacing must permit of observation by class and teacher, and this makes it necessary to provide for careful class arrangement on the floor. It is unnecessary to spend time drilling in opening order, even though the execution is somewhat ragged. The most important thing to consider, especially on a cold day, is to get the class *warmed up* and the lesson started as quickly as possible. The preliminary part of the lesson i.e., alignment, counting off, opening order and straightening lines, may all be done during the preliminary walking and running. Prior to opening order, a class has numbered off by two's, three's, four's, or five's.

Opening order may be taken:
(a) By side steps, or by turns and march steps forward from one or more files brought to the desired anterior-posterior alignment on the floor.
(b) By walking or running from the rear of the room to previously indicated positions.

The following diagrams illustrate a variety of ways of opening order by the second method:

1. *Opening from one file to make three*
   Class numbered by three's

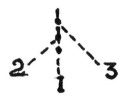

Signal: "Two's to the right, three's to the left, opening out—go!"

2. *Opening from one file to make five*

Class numbered by five's

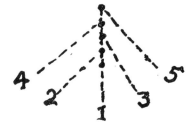

Signal: "Spreading out—two's and four's to the right —three's and five's to the left—go!"

3. *Opening from two files to make six*

Class numbered by three's

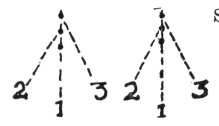

Signal: "Down center in two files—two's to the right—three's to the left—spreading out —go!"

4. *Opening from one or two files to make seven*

Class numbered by seven's

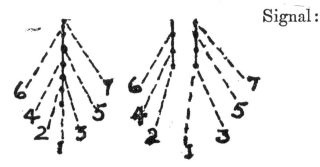

Signal: "Spreading out — two's, four's, a n d six's to the right, three's, five's and seven's to the left —go!"

5. *"Sunburst." Opening from two files to make four*
Class in double file formation numbered off by two's

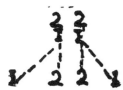

Signal: (after explanation) "Sunburst, open out—go!"

6. *"Fan." Opening from files of four*
Class does not necessarily need to be numbered

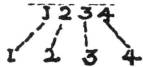

Signal: (As class forms four's at back of room) "Spreading out—go!"

7. (a) *"Spiral." Opening from files of four*
Class does not necessarily need to be numbered

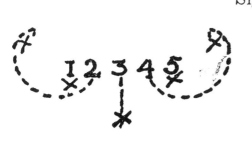

Signal: "Two inside files 'spiral out' with 6 (8) steps and turn; —outside files one side step—on 5 (7) counts—go!"

(b) *"Spiral." Opening from files of five*
Class does not necessarily need to be numbered

Signal: (As class forms five's at back of room) "Center file three steps forward,—inside files 'spiral' outward five (or seven) steps and back of outside files—go!"

8. *Opening from one file to make nine*

Class in column of three's numbered off by three's

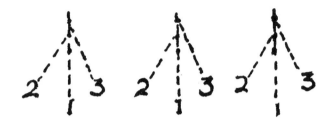

Signal: "Down the center in three files,
two's to the right, three's to the
left—spreading out—go!"

CHAPTER IV

PROGRESSION AND ADAPTATION

"Lacking the element of progression, no work can be of much educational value. Nor can pupils be expected to remain interested for any length of time in work in which they find nothing further to learn, or in which their growing strength and ability are not constantly given full scope, are not put to new and increasingly difficult tests." [1]

FACTORS CONTROLLING RATE OF PROGRESSION

These are obviously the (1) Environmental conditions under which the work is given, and (2) The type and capacity of a class.

Both these factors, including time allotment, will be operative in determining the length of the activity period, and the number of periods in a course.

1. *Environmental Factors*

In giving gymnastic work, it is important to consider climatic conditions as well as the immediate environment. First, the exercise room may be inadequate as to size and condition; the floor may be of such a nature as to exclude all exercises taken in a lying or sitting position; there may be no facilities for stall-bar exercises; it may be impossible to take a shower bath after

[1] Skarstrom, W., "Gymnastic Teaching," p. 131, Am. P. E. Assn.

a lesson; or a class may be required to return immediately to a class room upon the finish of a lesson. Second, the climate or temperature may vary, and work may have to be done in a warm, humid, or cold room. These factors will largely determine the selection, adaptation, and progression of exercises.

2. *Type and Capacity of a Class*

Lessons planned for children, women and men will differ regarding selection, duration and intensity of the activity. Work must be planned to meet the needs of the average, or really of the "mean deviation," of the class. It can quite rightly be argued that people in different spheres of life, of different sex and different occupations react differently to daily routine, but experience in teaching leads one to believe that individuals in any one group, are sufficiently alike to allow the teacher to set up a general scheme for the foundation work of bodily development. Very atypical individuals should, of course, be given individual work suited to their particular needs.

ADAPTATION FOR ELEMENTARY GRADES

Those teachers who have had actual experience in elementary schools will best be able to adapt this type of activity to their own situations. It is necessary, however, to understand the *material, aim and scope* of Fundamental Gymnastics before attempting the problem, if the outcome is to be satisfactory. When a child enters school and sits for long hours at a desk, the flexibility common to childhood rapidly disappears. This is especially noticeable in the reduced range of movement possible in the shoulder and hip joints, and in the stiffening of the dorsal and lumbar spine.

Children of elementary school age are interested in those exercises which embody a "stunt" element, like *alternate knee stretching with help of hands,* or *squat sitting hop with alternate leg stretching sideways.* They are also intrigued by co-ordination exercises that are like "tricks" or "stunts," such as *jumping with double, single and alternate arm stretchings.* The rhythmical element in such activities also appeals to the child.

The work must be made simple, with enough repetition to insure satisfaction and joy in accomplishment. An informal method of presentation is advised. Below the 4th grade, it is suggested that work be presented only in story play form.

In a few instances, work in pairs has been quite successfully carried out, but it is the general opinion that this couple work is not suitable for children.

When it is necessary to use a schoolroom instead of a gymnasium, only those exercises should be selected as may be used in the small space between desks. Arm flinging is not possible unless the pupils are turned in such a manner that there is no danger of knocking their knuckles against the desks. In some cases, it might be possible to have the children take the exercises from a sitting position on their desks. No work has, as yet, been especially adapted to meet this situation, but the ingenuity of the teacher will help him to take advantage of such unfavorable conditions and make the best of them.

Lesson plans should be short,—possibly not more than 8 to 10 exercises, given in a 10 to 12 minute period, —and progression should be easy but steady.

In junior and senior high schools, work may be progressively harder, with emphasis still on self-testing and rhythm. Here, attention should definitely be paid to faulty posture and weak musculature. Plenty of trunk work, relieved by precipitant exercises, gives the hygienic and physiological reaction necessary. Progression should be gradual, and entirely dependent upon the capacity of the class. Lessons should be longer and include 20 to 25 exercises in 20 minutes. Caution must be exercised not to overdo or push a class beyond its strength. There must be observation to detect the slightest signs of fatigue, so that the action may be immediately changed to another part of the body, or all work stopped. A class should leave the floor in "high spirits,"—feeling refreshed and exhilarated and never "dog-tired." This is the teacher's problem, and a big one, but the use of the work for this, or any age, depends upon its rational solution.

In colleges and universities, gymnastic activities are usually part of the required work in the winter terms of the first two years. In point of hours, this amounts to two or three half-hour lessons a week over a period of 14 or 15 weeks. These lessons are usually crowded in between academic classes. The modern type of woman college student is usually slender, underweight, and muscularly relaxed but not flexible. She is keen, quick-witted and intolerant of that which seems valueless to her, and responds quickly to things that seem to her to have real value. If conditions were ideal, the student would have had her basic training before she reached college age. During her college years, she could then choose her favorite activities,—games, athletics or dancing,—since her physical activities could be directed to meet only recreational and hygienic needs. The girl of today, however, reaches college markedly undeveloped and physically unco-ordinated. Under existing conditions, therefore, the university or college must give her the training that should have been part of her earlier education.

Many teachers who have taught Fundamental Gymnastics in colleges have found that students are keenly interested in and, in many cases, elect this type of activity. In each situation, there must be careful and intelligent selection and adaptation of exercises best suited to the needs of the student.

ADAPTATIONS FOR Y.M.C.A. AND Y.W.C.A. CLASSES

In Y.M.C.A. and Y.W.C.A. classes the work must be given with the recreative element paramount. These groups are entirely voluntary, attendance dependent upon desire for vigorous activity, either for fun or for health reasons. The younger business girl is approximately the same age as the college student, but because of her irregular life, long hours of inactivity in her work, and often poor food at odd hours, she has gradually lost her robust health of high school days. She is, nevertheless, full of life and desirous of strenuous activity. The older business man (or woman) is growing stiff or stout as the case may be, and has lost much of his vitality because of the occupational demands made upon him.

All classes for business men and women do, and should, lack strict discipline and formality, and the activities should be taught more or less informally. Attendance in these classes is apt to be irregular, and thus a rational progression is retarded. Repetition of exercises, and a great deal of trunk work,—much of it given when the class is lying on the floor,—will be found advantageous. The work must not be too strenuous, and little attention need be paid to exact form and smooth, rhythmical changes. With older men (or women), the vigor and intensity of the work must be reduced, and much of the heavier work and hanging exercises modified and carefully selected. Only the simplest of co-ordinations should be used, and a minimum number of easy precipitant exercises. Progression, with this type of adult, should be very gradual, and the teacher's powers of observation and judgment must be continually exercised.

ADAPTATION FOR SPECIAL INDIVIDUALS

The field of usefulness for Fundamental Gymnastics in the corrective gymnasium has proven to be a very large one. The greatest reason in favor of this type of work is that, in a comparatively short time, the effort expended is rewarded by a noticeable improvement. Another reason is, that the pupil gets a real joy out of the exercise, and is more interested in it because he can see his own improvement in the execution of the exercises and in the results attained. Many of the exercises that were formerly given, when taken out of the class work and made into an individual program, seemed to lose the *fun element* and *play spirit* and often, to those physically handicapped, became dull and uninteresting, and a mere duty performed under doctor's orders. Mr. Bukh's work is more objective, and has, within each exercise, a definite goal for each individual, and a possibility of self-testing. It is this, together with resultant interest on the part of the individual, that makes this work so adaptable to the corrective program.

The teaching problem, in the busy corrective gymnasium, is simplified by the use of this type of work because the pupil takes more responsibility upon himself, and seems to get the "feeling" of the exercises easily. While it is impossible to preserve the continuity of the lesson plan, that is, one exercise following another in sequence as Fundamental Gymnastics are taught in a class, it is possible to plan the program in such a way that after the exercises are learned separately, they can be joined together in groups of three or four. This stimulates interest, and the pupil enjoys making the change of movement.

The necessity of making many adaptations and changes to fit individual cases is very important to consider, and this work lends itself to these adaptations in an interesting way to both pupil and teacher.

It has been noted, that the child does not have to do the exercises with technical perfection before the results are noticeable, for the effort expended on each lesson in doing it as well as it can be done, gives him the maximum benefit attainable at that time, and the progression in his ability to do the work better is measured by the improvement in his condition.

Fundamental Gymnastics can be admirably adapted to meet the needs in the typical cases of maladjustment, organic as well as structural, which present themselves as problems for individual attention.

It is possible to deal with postural cases in small groups, to correct poor posture habits, to free the tensed and tightened muscles, and relieve ligamentous tension around the joints. In the outstandingly weak muscle areas, the antagonistic muscles are over-contracted and tense, and after a balance has been attained by stretching these muscles, the equally important task of strengthening the weak musculature is undertaken. Such an all-round posture program, built up for use in the corrective gymnasium, is especially useful in handling group work, thus efficiently treating, as individuals, the greatest number of students in the minimum amount of time and with minimum instruction.

One of the most important phases of posture work is the treatment of weak foot musculature. Outstandingly strong work for the feet is obtained in the hopping, toe touching, heel raising and knee bending, and in the exercises for leg flexibility which stretch the tendon of Achilles. Most important of all, is the strengthening of the feet through gripping of the floor for balance and support in those exercises where the arms are used as the long levers of the body, in bringing about forceful stretchings, flingings, bendings, and twistings.

ADAPTATION FOR NORMAL SCHOOLS OF PHYSICAL EDUCATION

In normal schools of physical education for women, a student's natural aptitude for physical activity enables her to progress much more rapidly, and do much more complex and difficult work.

Since a thorough course in gymnastics is usually given in normal schools, it is possible to proceed at a rational rate of progression from the freshman to the senior year. If, however, because of an already overloaded curriculum, the time devoted to Fundamental Gymnastics must be limited to 1 or 2 years, it is advisable to give this activity during the first years of training. It must be remembered that this is basic work, and it should always be considered as such. It, therefore, is *primary* rather than *supplementary* material. In some situations, where Fundamental Gymnastics have been placed in the first years, much of the developmental training, so necessary in dancing, has been taken care of, and time saved for actual dancing.

When Fundamental Gymnastics are given in normal schools, it is imperative that a thorough theoretical course in teaching methods, and an intensive and exhaustive study of the principles underlying the use of material, should be given.

3. *General Principles in Progression*

There are certain general principles in progression from exercise to exercise within the lesson, and from lesson to lesson.

1. Within the lesson

   This consists of a gradual rise and fall in the output of energy, i.e., a regular increase of muscular work demanded during the lesson. The lesson begins with some light work which quickly brings all muscles into action. The heavier trunk work, and exercises demanding greater energy and co-ordination, should come in the latter half of the lesson after the muscles have sufficiently "warmed up" to take care of the extra demand put upon them.

2. From lesson to lesson the following principles must be kept in mind.

   (a) Perfection of familiar exercises.
   (b) Acquisition of new material.

PERFECTION OF FAMILIAR EXERCISES

Repeating familiar exercises which are intrinsically valuable is important from two standpoints:

(1) The increase in range and intensity through repetition, makes for greater perfection of movement, thereby giving a class the satisfaction and joy which comes from expansion of the ego when work is well done. Students can not only see, but feel, the improvement, and this is one of the greatest agents in holding interest in the work.

(2) The teacher can use this means as a check upon previous work, i.e., how far the work has progressed; is the class more flexible, stronger, quicker and more adept. The principle of "the old in the new" applies here. By a change in position of arms, the addition of an extra hop or a deep knee bend, or through increasing the difficulty of co-ordinations by changes in direction or sequence, the familiar work will constantly take on an added interest. The teacher must ever keep in mind the ultimate perfection of an exercise even though, for the time being, he has to put off the actual attainment of that perfection, and be satisfied with a mediocre execution,—remembering that it takes time and patience to bring about freedom in shoulders and hip joints, and to strengthen backs and abdominal muscles. At first, it is best not to "worry" a class with too much "correction." Admonitions and stimulations are valuable and must constantly be used but, too much criticism and stopping and re-

calling movements result in a loss in continuity of motion, and often is discouraging
to a class that is ready for action. It is better
to keep a spirit of camaraderie in the group,—
knowing there will be adequate opportunity
for repeating and perfecting an exercise in
succeeding lessons. Later, however, if perfection of movement is desired, there must be a
conscious effort on the part of the teacher and
individuals in the class to correct all minor
defects in execution.

ACQUISITION OF NEW MATERIAL

New and complex work must be carefully analyzed
and broken up into simple elements, and first taught
in that form. The following examples illustrate this
method of procedure.

Exercise (1) *Hopping w. alt. toe touching sideways
and forward w. opp. arm stretching
sideways and forward.*

(a) Jump in place.
(b) Wing standing hopping w.
alt. toe touching sideways.
(c) Wing standing hopping w.
alt. toe touching forward.
(d) Wing standing hopping w.
alt. toe touching sideways
and forward.
(e) Arm bending and stretching
sideways (combined with
b.)
(f) Arm bending and stretching
forward (combined with c.).

(g) Alt. arm bending and stretching sideways.

(h) Alt. arm bending and stretching forward.

(i) Alt. arm bending and stretching sideways and forward. (combined with d.).

Exercise (2) *Neck stride bow standing trunk springing alternating with trunk stretching forward (or back stretching).*

(a) Trunk bending downward to grasp ankles.

(b) Grasp stride bow standing trunk springing.

(c) Stride angle standing trunk springing.

(d) Neck stride angle standing trunk springing.

(e) Neck stride angle standing trunk stretching forward.

The psychological principle of "the old in the new" must be applied in working out a satisfactory progression. There must be just enough of the *old* in each exercise to interest and appeal, and then the *new* element will be an added stimulation.

Often, to impose a new and difficult exercise, quite out of logical progression, "wakes up" a class and shows it how much there is yet ahead to master.

3. In planning a course of gymnastic lessons, possibly thirty in all, it has been found helpful, particularly with Fundamental Gymnastics, to work backward from a final (30th) lesson, or from the 15th lesson. After the first few lessons, which are planned as preliminary

tests of the condition of the class with regard to flexibility, strength and agility, the teacher has a mental picture of the probable improvement he can expect by the 15th and 30th period. He then prepares the median and final lessons, not with the fixed idea of reaching these in every particular, but as guides in the planning of intermediate lessons. To be more explicit he

(1) Makes a skeletal outline for the 30 lessons.
(2) Fills in the tentatively complete 15th and 30th lessons.
(3) Breaks up these 2 lessons into their elements.
(4) Indicates on the outline, those points (lessons) where new elements or special combinations of elements should be introduced.

It is not necessary to follow this method, but some such scheme is desirable if progression is to be logical and normally rapid.

As progression is made from lesson to lesson and from exercise to exercise, greater unison and uniformity of work may be expected. As the work is more or less individualized, the appearance of the class will be ragged and uneven, for everyone is working in his own rhythm and at his own speed. This is bound to be so because of individual variation in range and freedom, but as the work progresses and the tension and constriction in joints and muscles is gradually overcome, an almost perfect class unison will develop out of these many rhythms.

4. *Speed*

In beginner's classes the speed of exercises should be faster than in advanced classes. This is particularly true with regard to flexibility movements where the weight leverage of the body is a factor. Thus, arm flinging taken without tension, at a rapid speed, will more readily and effectively overcome ligamentous tension than at a slow one. The same is true of a quick deep knee bending where the body weight increases the force.

In a beginner's class, there will be a wide range of individual difference in flexibility, particularly in the shoulder girdle. In *arm flinging* if taken at too slow a speed, the less flexible students will, therefore, reach their maximum range in the fling, and begin the recoil of the movement before the more flexible, or they may attempt to hold the position and thereby lose the effect of the momentum of the exercise. Exercises for developing strength should be given at a comparatively slow speed, but even here it will be found advantageous to increase the rate slightly until the class has attained a moderate degree of strength. In *slow alternate deep knee bending,* for example, a weak class will be able to execute the exercise with less effort if the speed is not too slow. Movements must be carefully studied with regard to the rate of speed at which the exercises can be done most effectively.

5. *Rhythm*

Every individual has a natural rhythm at which he works most efficiently. This fact complicates the setting of a fixed rhythm and involves adjustment of speed to meet the average ability of a class. To do this, the rhythm set by the freest members of the group must be decreased, and the slow phlegmatic individuals must be urged to increase their rhythm. This, for a time, may upset their co-ordination and bring on fatigue too quickly, but as soon as they adjust to the more rapid rate, more efficient work will be done.

Many exercises in Fundamental Gymnastics involve both an *even* and *uneven* rhythm. Not only does this apply to consecutive exercises, but to parts of the same exercise. At first, it will be advisable to keep the movements as even as possible, but later, the mastery of a difficult, uneven rhythm, will be stimulating and satisfying.

In beginner's classes, it is not necessary to go from exercise to exercise without stopping. Separate exercises may be taught with a stop after each one. Later, as a class progresses, many rhythmical changes from one exercise to another may be made. As has been previously stated, progression in rhythm, in non-definite work, should be from a faster to a slower rhythm.

6. *Specific Principles in Progression*

Progression is measured by the following devices:

(a) Narrowing the base: exercises done with a broad base are considered easier because much of the balance element is eliminated.

(b) Raising the center of gravity: where the trunk exercises involve arm positions, raising the center of gravity, through changing these positions, increases the difficulty of the exercise.

(c) Fixation of parts of the body: through the selection of starting positions, parts of the body not involved in the exercise are fixed, thereby localizing the movement i.e., it is easier for a class to take a correct chest lifting from *back clasp knee bow sitting* than from the *erect standing* position.

(d) Isolation of parts to be moved: this makes for simplicity in the exercise and localizes the desired action, e.g., *hand knee standing trunk twisting with arm flinging.*

(e) Choice of starting positions involving restricted joint action: e.g., exercises taken from *long sitting* position are difficult for a stiff class.

(f) Increase in number of parts of the body moved: e.g., *chest lifting* from *arm side back lying* is easier than *arm, leg and chest lifting* from the same starting position.

(g) Increase in speed: there is less muscular resistance when a movement is taken at a comparatively rapid rate of speed.

(h) Increase in weight leverage: when the weight of the body increases the force and range of the movement e.g., *hand squat sitting knee stretching with trunk springing,* the exercise is stronger and more effective than *hand squat sitting knee stretching.*

CHAPTER V

A. ARM POSITIONS

1. *Wing (hip) standing:* Hands placed on hips, hands low, wrists relaxed.
   Signal: "Hands on hips—place!"

2. *Bend standing:* Elbows completely flexed without tension, finger tips lightly touching shoulders.
   Signal: "Arms—bend!"

3. *Neck standing:* Hands placed at back of neck.
   Signal: "Hands on neck—place!"

4. *Top standing:* Finger tips touching on top of head.
   Signal: "Hands on head—place!"

5. *Stretch standing:* Arms extended vertically upward, palms facing.
   Signal: (a) "Arms upward—stretch!" (through bend standing) or
   (b) "Arm raising forward—(sideways) upward—one!" or
   (c) "Arms forward—(sideways) upward—raise!"

6. *Arm side standing:* Arms raised horizontally sideways.
   Signal: (a) "Arms sideways — s t r e t c h !" (through bend standing) or

[1] *Note*—See page 131.

51

(b) "Arms sideways—raise!" or

(c) "Arm raising sideways—one!"

7. *Fold standing:* Arms in horizontal plane, elbows completely flexed at shoulder height, wrists straight without tension.

Signal: "Arms forward—bend!"

8. *Reach standing:* Arms raised horizontally forward, palms facing.

Signal: (a) "Arms forward — s t r e t c h ! "
        (through bend standing) or

(b) "Arm raising forward—cne!" or

(c) "Arms forward—raise!"

9. *Drag standing:* Arms stretched downward and backward.

Signal: "Arms backward—raise!"

10. *Ring standing:* Arms curved in ring over head, fingers extended and tips touching.

Signal: "Arms in ring over head—place!"

11. *Fly standing:* Arms raised diagonally upward over head. (In rhythmical work, fingers are curled and palms forward.)

Signal: (a) "Arms diagonally sideways-upward—raise!" or

(b) "Arms diagonally sideways-upward — stretch!" (through bend standing) or

(c) "Arms diagonally sideways-upward—fling!"

12. *"S" standing:* One arm in half ring over head, the other raised sideways with elbow completely flexed and hand placed close under arm pit. Wrist may be

straight with hand clenched, or heel of hand (fingers curled under), may be pressed against side of chest.

Signal: "Arms in 'S'—place!"

13. *Cross standing:* Arms crossed low in front of body.

Signal: (a) "Arms in cross—place!" or
(b) "Arms—cross!"

14. *Back clasp standing:* Hands locked low behind back.

Signal: "Hands backward—clasp!"

B. LEG POSITIONS

15. *Erect standing:* Position of perfect poise without tension.

Signal: (a) "With feet together—in position— stand!" or
(b) "With feet together — stand — erect!"

16. *Toe standing:* Heels raised, weight on toes.

Signal: (a) "Heels—raise!" or
(b) "On toes—stand!"

17. *Stride standing:* Feet placed two foot lengths apart, weight evenly distributed.

Signal: (a) "Left (right) foot sideways — place!" or
(b) "Feet sideways—place!" (This is executed with a jump.)

18. *Oblique standing:* One foot placed two foot lengths diagonally forward, weight evenly distributed.

Signal: "Left (right) foot outward—place!"

19. *Walk standing:* One foot placed two or three foot lengths directly in front of the other.

Signal: "Left (right) foot forward—place!"

20. *Oblique charge*

21. *Side lunge* } Not frequently used as starting positions.

22. *Forward charge*

23. *Squat sitting:* Trunk erect, knees completely flexed and separated.

Signal: "Knees deep—bend!"

24. *Hand squat sitting:* Same as in No. 23 except that hands are placed on floor in front of feet.

Signal: "With hands on floor—knees deep—bend!"

25. *Half knee standing:* Kneeling on one knee, the other foot placed forward, right angles in all joints.

Signal: (a) "On right (left) knee—down!" or
(b) "With left (right) foot forward—on right (left) knee—down!" or
(c) "With left (right) foot backward—on left (right) knee—down!"

26. *Knee standing:* Kneeling on both knees, right angles between thighs and legs.

Signal: "On knees—down!" (From erect standing always executed through squat sitting.)

27. *Knee sitting:* Kneeling (sitting on heels) trunk erect, ankles extended.

Signal: (From knee standing) "On heels—sit!"

28. *Half hook standing:* Standing on one leg, other

leg bent at knee, with right angles at hip and knee joints.

Signal: "Left (right) knee—lift!"

29. *Half hook lying:* Lying on back, position of legs the same as in No. 28.

Signal: "Left (right) knee—lift!"

30. *Half knee stride standing:* Kneeling on one knee, other leg stretched sideways.

Signal: (From knee standing) "Left (right) leg sideways—stretch!"

31. *Half squat stride sitting:* One knee in squat sitting, the other leg extended directly sideways.

Signal: (a) (From stride position) "Right (left) knee deep—bend!" or
(b) (From hand squat sitting) "Left (right) leg sideways—stretch!" or
(c) "With deep bending of left (right) knee, right (left) leg sideways—stretch!"

32. *Hurdle sitting:* Sitting with one leg stretched forward, other leg backward with knee bent, right angles in all joints, one hand grasping outside of forward foot, other hand grasping inside of rear foot.

Signal: "With left foot forward and right foot backward—in hurdle position—sit!"

33. *Hand knee standing:* Standing on hands and knees, trunk horizontal.

Signal: "On hands and knees—down!" or "stand!"

34. *Hook sitting:* Sitting on floor with knees bent and feet together.

Signal: "To hook sitting—down!"

35. *Cross sitting:* Sitting on floor, knees bent and feet crossed.

Signal: "To cross sitting—down!"

36. *Long sitting:* Sitting on floor, legs together and extended straight forward.

Signal: "To long sitting—down!"

C. TRUNK *POSITIONS*

37. *Hand foot lying:* Body extended and supported on hands and toes.

Signal: (a) "To hand foot lying—one!"—
"Two!" or

(b) "To hand foot lying—down!"

38. *Side hand foot lying:* Body extended and supported on one hand and outer edge of one foot with side of body toward floor.

Signal: "To side hand foot lying—one!"—
"Two!"—"Three!"

From hand foot lying on "Three" the body is turned to rest on one hand.

39. *Hand standing:* Standing on hands with or without support.

Signal: "On hands—up!"

40. *Back lying:* Body supine.

Signal: "On backs—down!"

41. *Angle standing:* Trunk bent forward at right angle from hips.

Signal: "Trunk forward—bend!"

42. *Bow standing:* Trunk bent downward as far as possible.

      Signal: (a) "Trunk bending downward—one!"
              or
            (b) "Trunk downward—bend!"

43. *Twist standing:* Trunk twisted to right or left.
      Signal: "To the left (right)—twist!"

44. *Front lying:* Body resting on floor, face down, hands under forehead.

      Signal: "To front lying—down!"

D. STALL BAR POSITIONS

45. *Hanging:* Hands grasping top bar, body hanging in stretch position.

      Signal: "With back against stall bars—from top
           bar—hang!"

46. *Bend hanging:* Hands grasping top bar, arms bent at right angles, body hanging with back against stall bars.

      Signal: "With arms bent at right angles—on
           top bar—hang!"

47. *Bow hanging:* Hanging, back to or facing stall bars, feet supported on same bar with hands.

      Signal: (From hanging position) "Feet on bar
           with hands—place!"

48. *Opposite arch hanging:* [2] Hands grasping bar high overhead, toes touching floor short distance backward. Chest is against bars, arms and legs are straight.

---

[2] This position is of questionable value except possibly for men with very strong back and abdominal muscles.

Signal: "Grasping bar overhead, in arch position—hang!"

49. *Angle hanging:* Low hanging, back and hips against stall bars, knees extended, heels resting on floor.

Signal: "Grasping bars shoulder height, knees deep—bend!" "Legs forward—stretch!"

50. *Opposite stride angle hanging:* Low hanging facing stall bars, hands wide apart and feet in stride position on bars, right angle at hips.

Signal: "With hands and feet wide on low bar—hang!"

CHAPTER VI

Flexibility is that condition of suppleness brought about by an adequate joint mobility and an accurate muscle action. The most complete motion desired in any joint may be secured through the use of such exercises as overcome all resistance in antagonistic muscle groups, through stretching and elongating muscles that are tense. When an exercise is not artificially inhibited, but is taken rhythmically and with vigorous momentum, such force, increased by the weight of the body or parts of the body, brings about complete joint mobility.

A. LEGS AND HIP JOINTS

1. *Opposite grasp toe standing quick deep knee bending and stretching in one count:* Executed in two's, facing with double hand grasp, or singly at stall bars or boom.

> Signal: "With double hand grasp in two's— stand!" "Heels—raise!" "Deep knee bending and stretching—one! (or begin)!"

2. *Opposite grasp standing quick heel raising and deep knee bending:* Executed in two's, facing with double hand-grasp.

> Signal: "Quick heel raising and deep knee bending—begin!"

[1] *Note*—See page 131.

59

3. *Wing standing quick heel raising and deep knee bending.*

Signal: (Name movement)—"begin!"

4. *Hand squat sitting hop with alternate leg stretching sideways:* The knee and ankle joint of the extended leg should be completely stretched. This exercise may also be executed—(a) Without the hop (b) In two's facing with double hand grasp.

Signal: (Name movement)—"begin!"

5. *Hand squat sitting jump with double leg stretching sideways (and backward).*[2] See illustration 5.

Signal: (Name movement)—"begin!"

6. *Opposite grasp squat sitting hop with alternate leg stretching forward.*

Signal: (Name movement)—"begin!"

7. *Jump between squat sitting and stride standing:* The hands may be supported on the knees in the squat position and changed to 'bend' or 'arm side' position as the hop is taken.

Signal: (Name movement)—"begin!"

8. *(Stall bars) Opposite grasp squat sitting spring to a squat sitting position on low bar:* In making the springs from the floor to the bar and from the bar to the floor, the body is extended with the head and chest held high.

Signal: "Spring to squat sitting on low bar— begin!"

---

[2] Boys' exercise.

E. LEGS, HIP JOINTS, AND LOWER BACK

The following exercises tend to stretch the usually over-shortened hamstring muscles. This stretching is accomplished in two ways (1) by applying pressure on the knee and forcing a complete straightening of the joint and (2) by strong downward bendings of the trunk (or 'trunk springing').[3] This downward bending straightens the lower back as well as stretches the hamstrings, providing the knees are kept straight. In those exercises involving flexion of the ankle, the stretching of the tendon of Achilles is a contributing factor in the correction of weak arches.

9. *Hand squat sitting knee stretching:* The hands are kept on or as near the floor as possible while the knees are being stretched.

> Signal: "With hands on floor knees deep— bend!" "Knees—stretch!"

10. *Trunk bending downward to grasp ankles.*

> Signal: "To grasp ankles, trunk downward— bend!" "Upward—raise!"

11. *Half grasp stride bow standing trunk springing:* Executed with one hand grasping the ankle on the same side, and the free arm hanging in a relaxed position.

> Signal: "Grasping left (right) ankle, trunk springing—begin!"

12. *Grasp stride bow standing trunk springing:* For girls the stride position should be narrowed.

> Signal: (From stride standing position) "Grasping ankles, trunk springing—begin!"

[3] Trunk springing—see Definitions and Explanations in Appendix.

13. *Long sitting trunk bending forward to grasp feet:*
This exercise may also be taken facing and with feet
against the stall bars. In bending forward the hands
grasp a low bar instead of the feet or ankles.

Signal: "To grasp feet or ankles, trunk forward
—bend!" "Upward—raise!"

14. *Grasp long bow sitting leg lifting with help of
hands:* During the exercise the knees must be kept completely extended, and the head and chest should be held
high.

Signal: (From starting position) "Leg (or heel)
lifting—begin!"

15. *Half knee standing trunk bending forward with
straightening of forward knee:* As the trunk is bent
and the forward knee straightened, the body drops to
a sitting position on the heel of the rear foot (ankle
extended). Both hands may be placed on the floor on
either side of the forward foot, or the forward foot may
be grasped by one or both hands.

Signal: (a) "Trunk   bending   forward   with
straightening of forward knee—
one!" "Trunk raising—two!" or
(b) "With   straightening   of   forward
knee, trunk forward—bend!" "Upward—raise!"

16. *Hurdle sitting trunk bending forward:* The
hand grasping the forward foot pulls the body forward
and downward, while the hand grasping the rear foot
lifts it clear of the floor, the toe pointed obliquely upward. Instead of relaxing after the movement, the forward foot may be lifted as the trunk is raised, thus
bringing about a strong stretching of the hamstrings.

Signal: (From starting position) "Trunk forward—bend!"

17. *Back lying single (or alternate) knee lifting and stretching with help of hands:* From the starting position, the left (right) knee is lifted, the right (left) hand grasps the foot, while the opposite hand is placed on the left (right) knee. Pressure is exerted on the knee as it is stretched.

Signal: (a) "Grasping foot and knee, left (right) knee—lift!" "Stretch!" "Bend!" "Stretch!" "Bend!" "Replace!" or

(b) "Knee stretching with help of hands—begin!"

18. *Alternate knee lifting and stretching with help of hands:* Executed and commanded as No. 17.

19. *(Stall Bars) Grasp bow standing arm bending:*

Signal: "Hand traveling downward on bars—go!"

"Arms—bend!" "Relax!"

20. *(Stall Bars) Grasp foot support bow lying knee stretching:* The knee stretching can be executed singly or together.

Signal: "On back with hands and feet supported on low bar—down!" "Knees—stretch!" "Relax!"

21. *(Stall Bars) Bow hanging foot support knee stretching:* Can be executed from hanging position or from angle hanging position with or without help.

Signal: "To bow hanging—up!" "Knees—Stretch!" "Relax!" "Slowly—sink!"

22. *Neck stride angle standing trunk springing:*
The work is executed by deep rhythmical springs from
the hip joints. It is possible that at the end of each bending the abdominal muscles exert a quick downward pull.

> Signal: (For starting position) "Hands on neck
> and left foot sideways—place!" "Trunk
> forward—bend!"
> (For movement) "Trunk springing—
> begin!"

23. *Hand squat sitting knee stretching with trunk
springing:* The work is executed rhythmically. As the
knees are stretched the trunk is slightly raised and then
swung downward toward the legs. The weight of the
trunk forces a complete straightening of the lower back,
and stretching of the hamstrings.

> Signal: (Name movement)—"begin!"

24. *Long sitting trunk springing with help:* Executed with helper who stands either in front of or behind his partner, and increases the deep rhythmical
bendings by a gentle pressure just below the shoulder
blades.

> Signal: (Name movement)—"begin!"

25. *(Stall Bars) Opposite grasp half leg high standing trunk bending forward:* The hands grasp a bar at
about head height and one leg is lifted as high as possible and supported against the stall bars. The body is
then pulled forward until the trunk and head are
brought near to the forcefully straightened knee.

> Signal: (From starting position) "Trunk for-
> ward—bend!" "Relax!"

26. *(Stall Bars) Opposite hurdle hanging, trunk*

bending forward: [4] From a *grasp squat sitting* position on the second or third bar, one leg is raised between the arms to a stretched position high over the head.

Signal: (From starting position) "Trunk forward—bend!" "Relax!"

27. *Grasp half angle lying trunk bending forward:* Both hands grasp the ankle of the leg that is raised to an angle of 45°. Executed in the same manner as No. 25.

Signal: (From starting position) "Trunk forward—bend!" "Relax!"

28. *Grasp half leg forward standing trunk bending forward:* Executed and commanded the same as No. 27.

C. ARMS AND SHOULDER GIRDLE

The arms, in *flingings, circlings,* and *stretchings,* are the agents that free the shoulder girdle through a stretching of the chest muscles, and the overcoming of ligamentous tension in the joints. In arm flingings, the counteraction of the trunk, together with the force of the movement, increases the stretching of the pectorals and is a big factor in overcoming the fixed and exaggerated convexity of the dorsal spine. [5]

29. *Half wing stride standing single arm circling:* The movement should be rapid and vigorous, and the trunk inclined slightly away from the circling arm. The arm circlings should be taken in the anterior-posterior plane with the fist clenched and the elbow extended. This exercise may also be executed in a *stride standing* position with *double arm circling.*

Signal: (Name movement)—"begin!"

[4] Boys' Exercise.
[5] See Section D. Neck and Upper back.

30. *Stride standing arm flinging between cross and fly:* Executed in free rhythmical flings, starting with arms crossed low in front of the body and continued obliquely upward and backward to a strong backward stretched *fly* position. The exercise may be made stronger and more effective when combined with *heel raising.*

> Signal: (Name movement)—"begin!" or "Arm flinging—begin!"

31. *Stride angle standing arm flinging between cross and fly:* Executed and commanded in the same manner as No. 30, except that the trunk is bent forward at an angle of 45°.

32. *Long sitting arm flinging between cross and fly:* Executed and commanded in the same manner as for above two exercises.

33. *Stride standing arm flinging between fold and arm side:* During the exercise the elbows are forced back in the *fold* position, and flung backward as far as possible in the *arm side* position. The exercise can also be executed while walking forward and backward.

> Signal: (Name movement)—"begin!"

34. *Stride angle standing arm flinging between drag and stretch:* In this exercise, the counteraction of the trunk is very important. The exercise may be taken with one or more easy arm swings between each fling.

> Signal: (Name movement)—"begin!"

35. *Arm circling in opposite directions (one forward and one backward):*[6] The feet may be in a narrow

---

● See Exercise 141 and Illustration 35.

stride position and the arms are swung in opposite directions at the same time.

>Signal: "Arm circling, left forward and right backward—begin!"

36. *Alternate and double arm flinging forward upward:* Executed in *erect standing* (*long sitting*) (*hook sitting*) position. Various leg movements may be added:

>With single arm flinging—
>>(a) Alternate toe touching backward.
>>(b) Alternate leg flinging backward.
>With double arm flinging—
>>(c) Heel raising.
>Signal: "Alternate and double arm flinging forward-upward—begin!"

37. *Side opposite grasp stride twist standing arm swinging sideways upward:* The chest must be kept lifted, the weight over the forward foot and the arms straight. This exercise is usually followed by *trunk springing,* or by *angle standing arm flinging between drag and stretch.*

>Signal: "In side opposite stride position— stand!" "Back to back—twist!" "With hand grasp, free arm flinging outward-upward—begin!"

38. *Long sitting arm circling with help:* May be executed with feet supported against the stall bars. The helper stands in a *forward charge* position with forward knee against his partner's back, and takes an over grasp hold along the inside of his upper arms. The *arm circling* is taken slowly forward and upward with a strong backward pull in the stretch position, then outward and downward.

Signal: (From starting position) (Name movement)—"begin!"

D. NECK AND UPPER BACK

The neck and upper back are both involved in most
of the exercises for each region respectively, and therefore work for the two regions are treated together.

In many individuals the head is carried forward and
the cervical curve exaggerated. This is a common dis-
figurement which may result in actual deformity.
Closely connected with this condition, it is usual to find
a round upper back and flat chest.

In some of the neck exercises, it will be noted that a
forward bending of the head precedes a stretching of
the spine. When the sixth cervical vertebra is anterior
and the seventh prominent, a forward bending of the
head is given to force the vertebrae into alignment. This
is immediately followed by a strong *chest lifting,* which
brings about an over extension of the spine and
straightens the cervical and dorsal regions, as well as
strengthens the muscles which hold the head and neck
in correct position upon the shoulders. (See exercises
for strength of Neck and Back.)

It has been proven that through persistent use of
such exercises, the prominence of the seventh cervical
may be quickly reduced.

In connection with these exercises, emphasis should
be placed on the importance of straightening the upper
back. In the dorsal region there is usually great stiffness with increased convexity. The muscles in this region cannot be properly developed because they are in
a more or less stretched condition, due to tight chest
muscles and to the lack of flexibility in the dorsal region. The over-contracted chest muscles pull the shoul-

ders forward, increasing the condition of round back and fixing the exaggerated convexity of the dorsal spine. The stretching of these muscles, as in *arm flinging,* combined with work for flexibility of the dorsal region, frees the shoulder girdle and brings about that mechanical condition which is necessary before strengthening and kinesthetic postural training can be successfully given.

39. *Head turning:* Executed by turning the head slowly and as far as possible to either side.
    Signal: "Head to the left—turn!" or
        "Head turning left and right in rhythm —begin!"

40. *Head bending forward and backward:* The bending forward should be done as high, and the bending backward as low, in the neck as possible.
    Signal: "Head forward—bend!" "Backward— bend!" or
        "Head bending forward and backward in rhythm—begin!"

41. *Head bending sideways:* Executed slowly directly to the side, and as deeply as possible.
    Signal: "Head to the left—bend!" "To the right—bend!" or
        "Head bending left and right—begin!"

42. *Head circling:* Executed slowly in a large circle.
    Signal: "Head circling to the left or right— begin!"

NOTE: In the last four exercises, it is essential to have the upper back in as stretched and straight a position as possible. For beginners, it is advisable to take, as a starting position, *grasp hook sitting* (hands around knees). The back is stretched and the body pulled close to the knees. The *head turning* or *bending* or *circling* is more effective from this position.

43. *(Stall Bars) Opposite grasp stride angle standing back stretching with help:* Executed in a stride position with feet on the floor, the body bent forward at right angles, and the arms supported on the bars (in a stretched position). The helper stands between his partner's arms, with his back against the bars, and with his hands on his partner's shoulder blades presses downward with an easy springing motion.
Signal: (Name movement)—"begin!"

44. *(Stall Bars) Stretch grasp hook lying chest lifting with help:* Executed in the *hook lying* position, hands grasping the third or fourth bar. The helper stands in a *stride position,* with his feet gripping his partner's hips, and his hands under his partner's shoulder blades. In this position the helper rhythmically works the shoulder region up and down, lifting the trunk as high as possible.
The exercise is more difficult when taken from a *back lying* position.
Signal: "Trunk—lift!" "Relax!" or
"Chest lifting with help—begin!"

45. *(Stall Bars) Stretch grasp knee standing back stretching with help:* Executed with back against the stall bars in a half-sitting, half-kneeling position, with the hands grasping a bar high over head. The helper faces his partner,—feet between partner's knees,—own knees gently pressing partner's thighs, and hands on his shoulder blades. The helper leans backward, throw-

ing the weight of his body into the movement, as he easily and rhythmically pulls his partner's body forward and slightly downward.

Signal: "Back stretching with help—begin!"

46. *(Stall Bars) Opposite stride angle hanging back stretching with or without help:* The helper stands behind his partner, and with his hands on partner's shoulder blades, gently presses downward with an easy springing motion.

Signal: (Name movement)—"begin!"

47. *Opposite foot support long sitting back stretching with help:* Executed in *long sitting* position with feet against low stall bar (or the feet of another person sitting opposite). The hands are clasped behind helper's neck or round his waist. The helper stands in a *charge* position behind his partner, hands on his own forward knee, and palms against his partner's back in the dorsal region. The work is performed as the helper bends his knee forward, and at the same time extends his trunk upward and backward, as he bends his rear knee. The exercise is continued rhythmically. This stretches the chest and arms, and arches the dorsal region. *Trunk springing with help* should be given as a compensatory exercise.

Signal: (From starting position) (Name movement)—"begin!"

48. *(Stall Bars) Hanging back stretching with shoulder support or angle hanging span bending with shoulder support:* Executed from *angle hanging* position on the stall bars. The performer executes as good a *span bending* as possible and, on the signal "support," the helper steps under his partner, and by placing his shoulders against the performer's shoulders, lifts him easily from the floor. There should be contact only at the shoulders, as the helper swings his partner in a rhythmical movement.

> Signal: (From starting position) "Span bending—one!" "Supporting p a r t n e r— two!"

49. *(Stall Bars) Hanging back stretching with foot support or angle hanging span bending with foot support:* [7] Executed in the same manner as No. 48, except that the helper lies on his back with hands grasping low bar, and feet supported (knees bent) against his partner's shoulders. On the signal, "stretch," the helper slowly straightens his knees and lifts his partner to a strong *arch hanging* position.

> Signal: "Span bending — one!" "Supporting partner—knees stretch!"

50. *(Stall Bars) Opposite stretch grasp knee bow sitting and back stretching with help:* [8] Executed with helper. The performer sits on his heels, facing the stall bars. His arms are straight and his hands grasp the fourth or fifth bar. The helper stands with his back to the stall bars and between his partner's arms, and gives a gentle rhythmical pressure in the shoulder region.

> Signal: (From starting position) "Back stretching—begin!"

51. *(Stall Bars) Stretch grasp hook sitting back stretching with help:* Executed in *hook sitting* position with lower back against stall bars, and with hands grasping high bar. The helper gives support, either with his feet placed between his partner's legs and his own knees bent outward, or standing outside his part-

[7] Boys' exercise.
[8] See picture for variation in method. Suitable only for boys.

ner's feet, exerting pressure knee against knee. In both cases the helper's object is to keep his partner's lower back close to the stall bars while he is pulling his partner's shoulders forward. The movement should be executed rhythmically.

> Signal: (From starting position) (Name movement)—"begin!"

52. *Back clasp front lying arm bending with back stretching:* In *front lying* position clasp hands around feet (knees bent). The bending of the arms produces a strong upper back stretching.

> Signal: (From starting position) "Arms—bend!" "Relax!"

E. LATERAL TRUNK

The work for flexibility of the side has to do most particularly with the lateral movements of the spinal column. These exercises affect the lumbar region, where the greatest movement naturally is found, but they should be given specifically for the dorsal region where the stiffness is greatest. While the anterior and posterior muscles of the trunk are those involved in twistings and bendings, it seems best to group the following exercises in a separate section. In the twistings and in the bendings which have to do with the approximation of the trunk to the legs in the lateral plane, the maximum range of movement is secured through the use of the arms as long levers, or for the purpose of applying localized pressure.

In this section, the twistings and bendings should at first be repeated several times to one side with a change to the opposite side on a given signal. Later they may be taken rhythmically from side to side.

53. *Half wing stride standing trunk twisting with single arm flinging:* The free arm is swung diagonally upward and backward as the twisting is taken. The arm is then swung downward and forward across the body continuing to the opposite shoulder and producing a small counter twist in the opposite direction.

> Signal: (From starting position) "Trunk twisting with single arm flinging—begin!"

54. *Stride standing trunk twisting with arm flinging from side to side:* Executed with alternate side twistings, allowing one arm to swing forcefully backward a little over shoulder height, while the other arm follows the movement across the chest to the shoulder. The chest should be lifted and the head turned to follow the movement of the straight arm.

> Signal: (Name movement)—"begin!"

55. *Stride angle-standing trunk twisting with arm flinging from side to side:* Executed and commanded like No. 54 except that in the starting position the trunk is bent forward.

56. *Hand knee standing trunk twisting with single (or alternate) arm flinging.*

> Signal: (Name movement)—"begin!"

57. *Hand stride foot lying trunk twisting with arm flinging.*

> Signal: (From starting position) (Name movement)—"begin!"

58. *Long stride foot support sitting trunk twisting with arm flinging from side to side.*

> Signal: (From starting position) (Name movement)—"begin!"

59. *Top stride standing side bending.*

    Signal: "Hands on top of head and feet side-ways—place!" "Side bending—begin!"

60. *"S" stride half toe standing side bending.*

    Signal: "With left toe touching sideways, arms in 'S'—place!" "Side bending—begin!"

61. *"S" stride standing side bending with (single heel raising or) opposite knee bending:* May be executed with various arm positions. The strong bending is always over the straight knee.

    Signal: (Name movement)—"begin!"

62. *Half knee stride standing, side bending:* Executed with hands on head or arms in "S" position.

    Signal: (From knee standing position)—"Arms in 'S' and left (right) foot sideways—place!" "Side bending—begin!"

63. *Top half squat stride sitting side bending:* Executed with the bending toward the straight knee. Various arm positions may be used.

    Signal: "With single deep knee bending, side bending—begin!"

64. *(Stall Bars) Side opposite foot support half standing side bending:* Executed with side to the stall bars and with inside foot supported on bar at a height halfway between knee and hip. The arms may be supported on the head or in "S" position. Several rhythmical bendings toward the stall bars should be followed by a strong compensatory bending to the other side.

    Signal: (From starting position)—"Side bending toward the bars—begin!"

65. *Hand side foot lying, hip raising:* This may be combined with quick trunk bending forward from back lying position.

> Signal: (From starting position) "Hips—lift!"
> "Relax!" or "Hip raising—begin!"

CHAPTER VII

EXERCISES FOR STRENGTH

In the following group of exercises the bendings and stretchings should be taken rhythmically, without sudden jerks or pauses, or in any position where the circulation to the active muscles might be restricted.

A. LEGS

66. *Wing standing slow heel raising and deep knee bending.*[1]

> Signal: (a) "Heels—raise!" "Knees deep—bend!" "Knees—stretch!" "Heels —sink!" or
>
> (b) (Name movement) "Slowly in rhythm—begin!"

67. *Stride standing slow alternate half knee bending.*[1]

> Signal: (From starting position) "Alternate slow half knee bending, in rhythm—begin!"

68. *Opposite grasp stride standing slow alternate deep knee bending:* The grasp may be single with the free hand placed on the hip or raised diagonally upward

---

[1] May be executed with various arm positions or combined with arm movements.

during the knee bending. This exercise may also be executed with the partners in—

> *Side opposite half grasp stride standing position:*
> (a) Facing in the same direction or
> (b) Facing in opposite directions.
> Signal: "Alternate slow deep knee bending, with the left (right)—begin!"

69. *Stride standing single knee bending and stretching pushing off:* [1] The knee bending preparatory to the strong extension and *push off* must be an easy one, an the landing should be light. A *side bending* may be added to this exercise, making it a lateral trunk move ment. In the bending, the trunk is inclined away fro the bent knee and toward the stretched knee.

> Signal: "*P*ushing off from left (right) foot— begin!"

70. *Stride standing slow alternate deep knee bending.* [1]

> Signal: (From starting position)
> (a) "Left (right) knee deep—bend!"
> "Stretch!" or
> (b) "Alternate slow deep knee bending in rhythm—begin!"

71. *Opposite half grasp stride standing slow alternate deep knee bending (with turn) and with opposite arm raising diagonally upward:* With left (right) hand grasp, the knee bending is taken to the left (right) side. Executed in two's, facing with single hand grasp.

> Signal: "Left (right) knee deep—bend!" "To opposite side—change!"

72. *Reach standing slow deep knee bending:* As the

left (right) leg is raised forward, the right (left) knee bends to a full *squat sitting* position. This exercise may also be executed in two's, facing, with double hand-grasp.

> Signal: "Arms and left (right) leg forward— raise!" "Right (left) knee deep—bend!" "Stretch!"

B. ARMS AND SHOULDER GIRDLE

It is not necessary or advisable to develop the same degree of strength in the arms of girls and women as for boys and men. For the latter, the successful execution of backflips, handsprings, and cartwheels is largely dependent upon arm strength. However, if many of the self-testing activities given to girls on the floor and apparatus are to be done efficiently and with satisfaction, the triceps muscles must receive more training than has until recently been considered necessary.

The biceps muscles are usually much stronger than the triceps and, therefore, the exercises in this section will deal principally with the development of the latter. The biceps are strengthened by their use in many of the exercises where the arms are involved.

73. *(Stall Bars) Opposite support ring stride standing arm bending and stretching.*

> Signal: (From starting position) "Arms— bend!" "Stretch!"

74. *(Stall Bars) Opposite stride standing arm springing pushing off from the stall bars.*

> Signal: (Name movement)—"begin!"

75. *Ring hand knee standing arm bending and stretching* (see illustration): During the bending, the elbows are moved outward to touch the floor. The bend-

ing may be alternated or combined with knee stretching. The exercise can be made stronger by placing the hands farther forward; or by supporting the weight on one arm with the free hand on the hip; or with one leg extended upward.

> Signal: "With right hand crossed over left—on hands and knees—down!" "Arms— bend!" "Stretch!"

76. *Ring hand stride angle standing arm bending and stretching:*[2] Executed and commanded like No. 75. Variations of the starting position may be:
>   (a) Hand foot lying
>   (b) Hand foot one half leg high lying.

77. *Knee standing arm springing pushing off from floor and arm flinging between cross and fly:* The arm springing pushes the body to a knee standing position, and is immediately followed by *arm flinging from cross to fly.* A strong counteraction of the trunk results from the forward fall of the trunk (to the next arm springing) before the arms have quite reached the *fly* position.

> Signal: (From starting position) "Arm springing from floor and arm flinging between cross and fly—begin!"

78. *Stride angle standing arm springing pushing from floor and trunk springing with hands on neck.*
> Signal: (Name movement)—"begin!"

79. *Stride front lying arm stretching with trunk lifting:*[2] The toes are bent under and the whole body is lifted during the movement.
> Signal: "Arms—stretch!"—"Bend!"

[2] Boys' Exercise.

80· *Hand standing arm bending with help.*[3] Helper may assist partner by supporting him at ankles or hips.

Signal: (From starting position) "Arms—bend!"—"Stretch!"

C. ARMS AND BACK

81. *(Stall Bars) Opposite stride angle hanging trunk lifting:* During the trunk lifting the elbows are raised as high as possible and the head (in line with the back) touches one bar lower than the hands.

Signal: "Arms—bend!"—"Stretch!"

82. *(Stall Bars) Stride angle hanging trunk lifting with help. "Wheelbarrow":* The helper stands between his partner's legs and lifts them as he would lift a wheelbarrow. During the trunk lifting the elbows are pushed backward and the trunk is forced forward.

Signal: "Arms—bend!" "Stretch!"

83. *(Stall Bars) Opposite arch hanging trunk lifting.*[3]

Signal: (From starting position, grasping bar h i g h o v e r head) "Arms—bend!" "Stretch!"

84. *(Stall Bars) Bend high hanging (feet supported) slow arm stretching:* The arm stretching may also be executed with the knees raised upward.

Signal: "Arms slowly—stretch!"

(To return to starting position) "With help of feet—up!"

85. *(Stall Bars) Opposite grasp bow sitting trunk*

---

[3] Boys' Exercise.

lifting: During the arm bending the elbows are lifted and held backward as far as possible.

> Signal: (For starting position) "With right (left) side to the stall bars in hook sitting—down!" "Grasping bar with right (left) hand (at head height) legs upward—swing!" (For movement) "Arms—bend!" "Relax!"

86. *(Stall Bars) Opposite bow hanging trunk lifting.*

> Signal: (For starting position on stall bars) "From opposite grasp squat sitting on low bar, feet up between the arms—place!" (For movement) "Arms—bend!" "Relax!"

87. *Opposite grasp foot support hook sitting alternate and double leg stretching and forward pulling of trunk:* The pulling of the trunk takes place after the legs are stretched (single as well as double). In single leg stretching, since partners are facing, the legs to be stretched cannot be indicated as "left" or "right." The signal must relate the stretching to some object or boundary of the room; e.g., stall bars, windows, clock.

> Signal: (a) "Legs toward (the stall bars)—stretch!"
> (b) "Toward (the clock) trunk—pull!"
> (c) "In opposite direction pull!" "Knees—bend!" (Repeat with other leg.)
> (d) "Both legs upward—stretch!"
> (e) "Toward (the clock) trunk—pull!" "In opposite direction—pull!"
> (f) "Legs—bend!"

*Back*88. *Opposite grasp stride long sitting trunk pulling forward:* Executed by quick changes from *back lying* to *bow sitting.*

> Signal: (From starting position) "Alternate forward pulling of trunk—begin!"

D. NECK AND BACK

89. *Arm side back lying head bending forward.*
> Signal: "Head forward—bend!" "Relax!"

90. *Grasp half hook lying head bending forward (alternating with chest lifting).*
> Signal: "Head f o r w a r d—bend!" "Relax!"
> ("Chest—Lift").

91. *Arm side back lying head and alternate knee lifting (alternating with chest lifting).*
> Signal: "Head and left (right) knee—upward
> —lift!" — "Relax!" "Chest — lift!"—
> "Relax!"

92. *Arm side front lying hip raising.*[4]
> Signal: "Hips lift!" "Relax!"

93. *(Stall Bars) Opposite neck hanging with support of helper.*[4]
> Signal: (Name movement)—"Up!" "Support!"

94. *Opposite foot support stride long sitting lifting of hips with support of helper:* The helper may give support at his partner's neck in either of two ways. (1) In *charge* position with his hands cupped on his forward knee. (2) In *reach·* (palms facing upward) *back lying position.* After the performer's body is raised

---

[4] Boys' Exercise.

to position, *arm bending and stretching* may be taken. Since the object of Exercises Nos. 93 and 94 is primarily to strengthen the neck muscles, the neck must be kept straight and the chin held in during the *hip lifting.*

> Signal: (From starting position) "Hips—lift!"
> "Relax!"

95. *Neck stride bow standing back stretching (trunk stretching forward):* In the starting position the back is relaxed and the elbows are dropped. During the *back stretching,* the elbows and shoulders are forced backward and upward as far as possible.

> Signal: "Hands on neck and left foot sideways
> —place!" "Trunk downward—bend!"
> "Trunk forward—stretch!" "Relax!"

96. *Neck long bow sitting chest lifting:* During the *chest lifting* the elbows are forced backward.

For variation the hands may grasp the feet in the starting position and be raised (through *bend*) to a *stretch* position as the chest is lifted.

> Signal: (From starting position)—"Chest—
> lift!" "Relax!"

97. *Grasp hook bow sitting chest lifting:* During the *chest lifting* the hands may be kept clasped about the knees or changed to a *low hand turning* outward, with finger tips touching the floor as far out to each side as possible.

> Signal: (From starting position) "Chest lifting
> with low hand turning—one!" "Two!"

98. *Back clasp knee bow sitting chest lifting:* Executed by slowly lifting the chest and strongly extending the neck and upper spine. In relaxing, the body is bent

forward with the forehead against the floor close to the knees.

> Signal: (From kneeling position) (For starting position) "Clasping hands behind the back, on heels—sit!"
>
> (For movement) "Chest—lift!" "Relax!"

ᛒ 99. *Chest lifting with low hand turning:* This exercise is most valuable for a person with a strong and flexible trunk. A beginner should place his hands over the abdomen to prevent a hollowing of the lower back. Each *chest lifting* may be followed by a compensatory *trunk bending downward*—to grasp ankles.

> Signal: "With low hand turning—chest—lift!" "Relax!"

ᛒ 100. *Front lying chest lifting with arm raising sideways:* To increase the difficulty of the exercise, the legs may be raised backward (with or without knee bending) as the arms are raised sideways.

> Signal: "Arms (legs) and chest—lift!"

ᛒ 101. *Arm side back lying chest lifting:* During the exercise the shoulders should be relaxed and the strong *chest lifting* aided by pressure of the head (chin in) against the floor.

> Signal: "Chest—lift!" "Relax!"

ᛒ 102. *Grasp half hook lying chest lifting.*
> Signal: "Chest—lift!" "Relax!"

103. *(Stall Bars) Stretch grasp hook lying chest lifting.*
> Signal: "Chest—lift!" "Relax!"

104. *(Stall Bars) Angle hanging span bending with help:* The performer stands with his back to the stall bars, grasping a bar at shoulder height. He bends his knees and extends his legs forward, keeping hips close to the bars and ankles relaxed. As the performer attempts to take a *span bending* position, the helper places one hand on his upper back and the other against his abdomen and gives slow, strong pressure upward and inward (with both hands), thus lifting his chest and bringing him into a correct position.

> Signal: "Span   bending—one!"   "Support—
> two!" "Relax!"

105. *(Stall Bars) Angle hanging span bending:* This exercise should not be attempted until the shoulder girdle is free and the back and abdomen strong. There should be no strain in reaching or holding the position.

In a perfect *span bend* the heels are raised, abdomen flat, chest lifted, chin in and head on a line with the arms. A standing, downward bending of trunk should always follow a *span bending* as a compensatory exercise.

> Signal: (From starting position) "Span bend-
> ing—one!" "Two!"

106. *(Stall Bars) Hand standing span bending.*[5]
> Signal: "Hand stand—one!" "Span bending—
> two!" "Replace!"

E. ABDOMEN

107. *Arm side back lying alternate and double high knee lifting:* Knee stretching may be added.
> Signal: "High   knee   lifting,   stretching   and
> slow sinking—in rhythm—begin!"

[5] Boys' Exercise.

108. *Opposite foot support back lying trunk bending forward:* Executed either with feet supported in stall bars or with legs locked with partner. The arms may be clasped in *ring* over head or crossed over chest.

> Signal: (From starting position) "Trunk bending forward—begin!"

109. *Arm side back lying slow trunk bending forward:* As the body is bent forward (chest leading) to grasp the feet, the arms aid the movement by pressing the palms against the floor.

> Signal: (From starting position) "Slow forward bending of trunk to grasp feet—one!" "Two!"

110. *Ring back lying trunk bending forward:* Executed in a quick rhythm. On the *forward bending,* the hands separate and slap the floor as far as possible beyond the feet.

> Signal: (Name movement)—"begin!"

111. *(Stall Bars) Opposite foot support back angle lying trunk bending forward to grasp stall bars:* Executed with heels resting on fourth or fifth bar and arms in ring over head or crossed over chest. *Arm bending* may be executed after grasping the bar.

> Signal: (From starting position) "Forward bending of trunk—one!" "Backward —two!"

112. *(Stall Bars) Hanging high knee lifting, stretching and slow sinking:* The exercise may be made more difficult by swinging the legs to *bow hanging* position, followed by *knee stretching* and *slow sinking.*

> Signal: (From starting position) (Name movement) "begin!"

113. *Stride front lying hip raising.*
      Signal: "Hips—raise!"—"Relax!"

114. *Stretch grasp standing alternate and double high knee lifting, stretching and slow sinking.*
      Signal: (Name movement)—"begin!"

115. *Arm side back lying trunk and leg raising upward.* (See illustration.)
      Signal: (Name movement)—"One!" "Two!"

116. *Opposite knee sitting trunk bending backward with support of helper:* The helper gives support during the exercise by exerting pressure on his partner's knees. As the performer bends backward, he gets support by sliding his hands outward along the floor. On the completion of the exercise the helper bends forward and his partner gives *trunk springing.*
      Signal: "Trunk   bending   backward — one!"
      "Trunk   raising — two!"   "T r u n k
      springing—begin!"

F. LATERAL TRUNK

117. *Hand side foot lying hip raising.* (See illustration 65.)
      Signal: "Hips lift!"—"Relax!"

118. *Neck back angle lying leg swinging from side to side with support of helper:* Executed with helper in *knee standing* position or in *stride angle standing* position, supporting his partner's elbows. The swing should be done slowly from side to side (right angle at hip joint). The helper, who gives strong support on the elbow opposite the direction of the movement, may

take single *arm bending* with free hand supported on hip.

> Signal: (From starting position) (a) "Leg swinging to the left—one!" "To the right—two!" or (b) "Slow leg swinging from side to side—begin!"

CHAPTER VIII

Exercises for Co-ordination

As all muscle groups in the body are antagonistically opposed to each other, relaxation or inhibition must be considered as important an active state of a muscle as contraction. If one group of muscles is stimulated to act, the opposing group must be inhibited or receive a stimulus to relax.

When the finely adjusted co-operation, or reciprocal innervation, is perfected, it results in great smoothness of movement, grace and skill.

The successful execution of any exercise involving arms or legs or trunk or a combination of all three, tests one's power of co-ordination and muscle sense but, it will be noted, that the exercises in this section deal particularly with arm and leg exercises of rather a simple nature. The unique manner of combining them gives them their peculiar interest and value. For example, the joining of a simple, three count leg movement with a simple two count arm movement; or a *circling* leg movement with a *stretching* arm movement; or a simple compound *arm stretching* movement where one arm is started one count before the other.

An exercise of this type gives a challenge similar to that found in self-testing activities and stunts.

It is advisable to keep these exercises quite simple, with no long and involved combinations which would presuppose much memorizing and *drilling*. After such exercises have been learned they have little value for co-ordination, but their repetition gives the same satisfaction experienced in doing a *stunt* after it has once been accomplished.

A. LEGS

119. *Jump in place:* Executed lightly on the balls of the feet, with good ankle action. The body is held erect without tension, the arms hanging free.
      Signal: "Small jumps in place—begin!"

120. *Alternate foot placing sideways.*
      Signal: (a) "Left (right) foot sideways—place!" or
              (b) "Alternate foot placing sideways —begin!"

121. *Alternate foot placing forward.*
      Signal: Same as for No. 120.

122. *Alternate foot placing obliquely forward.*
      Signal: Same as for No. 120.

NOTE: There is no great value in foot placings save as they give training in accuracy and in weight distribution.

123. *Alternate (or single) knee lifting.*
      Signal: "Alternate knee lifting—begin!"

124. *Easy heel raising and knee bending.*[1]
      Signal: (Name movement)—"Begin!"
            begin!"

125. *Toe touching:*[1] This exercise may be taken in all directions. The ankles should always be well extended.

[1] May be executed with various arm positions or combined with arm movements.

Signal: (a) "Toe touching to left (right)—
one!" "Two!" or
(b) "Toe touching sideways (forward)—begin!"

126. *Jump between stride standing and standing:*
Executed with hands supported on hips or with arms
swinging outward and upward to clap hands over head,
with one or more jumps between. Can also be done with
turns on the jumps. The exercise may be varied by
jumping twice (or more) in place and (or) by adding
a turn left or right on the last jump.

Signal: (a) (Name movement) — "Begin!"
or—
(b) "Jump with foot placing sideways
and together—begin!"

127. *Two hops with alternate leg flinging sideways:*[1] This exercise may be executed with any number of hops.

Signal: (Name movement)—"Begin!"

128. *Hop with alternate toe touching sideways:*[1]
This exercise may also be executed as—(a) Hop with
alternate toe touching forward—or (b) Hop with alternate toe touching sideways and forward—or (c) Hop
with alternate toe touching sideways and turning with
toe touching forward. (See Chapter IX, 16.)

129. *Two hops with alternate knee lifting:*[1] Opposite arm swinging forward with the knee lifting makes
an excellent combination.

Signal: (Name movement indicating desired
arm movements)—"Begin!"

130. *Jump and hop with alternate knee lifting.*
    Signal: (Name movement, indicating desired
        arm movements)—"Begin!"

131. *Three hops with alternate leg swinging in
circle:*[1] To start the exercise, place the right foot
under the heel of the left foot as the left foot is raised
forward and started on the swing.
    Signal: (Name movement)—"Begin!"

132. *Four hops with alternate leg swinging forward
and backward.*[1]
    Signal: (Name movement)—"Begin!"

133. *Four hops with alternate toe touching sideways
and knee lifting and toe touching forward and knee
lifting:*[1] On the first hop (on the right foot), place
the left toe sideways; on the second hop (on the right
foot), lift the left knee forward; on the third hop (on
the right foot), touch left toe forward; on the fourth
hop (on the right foot), lift the left knee and change
to the left foot with hop.
    Signal: (a) "Hop with toe touching sideways
            and forward and knee lifting—
            begin!" or
        (b) (Name movement) "in rhythm—
            begin!"

134. *Jump from squatt sitting to stride standing and
standing:* May be done with hands on hips or on knees
during deep knee bending position, and with hand clapping over head in the *stride* position.
    Signal: (Name movement)—"begin!"

135. *Alternate leg swinging forward and backward
with hand clapping:* The clap is taken (1) under the

knee of raised leg, (2) over head as the leg is swung backward, (3) behind the back as the feet come together. (3 counts.)

Signal: (Name movement)—"Begin!"

136. *Back angle lying double, single, or alternate bending and stretching of ankle and knee.*

Signal: (For starting position) "On back with feet high and knees straight—down!" (For movement on count) (a) "Ankles — bend!" "Knees — bend!" "Knees — stretch!" "Ankles—stretch!" or (b) (Name movement) "in rhythm—begin!"

137. *Front lying single, double or alternate bending and stretching of knee and ankle.*

Signal: (From starting position) "Front lying —down!"

(For movement) same as for No. 136.

B. ARMS

138. *Arm stretching:* Always taken through *bend* position. May be executed in one or more directions, with one or both arms. The *double arm stretching* may be made more difficult by starting and continuing the stretching of one arm one count ahead of the other.

Signal: (a) "Arms — bend!" (Name directions)—"stretch!" or

(b) "Arm stretching (in named directions and sequence)—"begin!"

139. *Arm placing:* May be executed singly or together, and by starting and continuing the placing of one arm one count ahead of the other.

Signal: (a) "Arms (in named position)—place!" or

(b) "Arm movements (in named directions and sequence)—in rhythm —begin!"

140. *Arm swinging.*
Signal: "Arm swinging (in named directions and sequence)—begin!"

141. *Arm circling:* May be double (in the same direction) or single in opposite directions.
Signal: (a) "Arm circling—begin!" or

(b) "Arm circling in opposite directions, one forward, one backward —begin!"

CHAPTER IX

A. COMBINED OR BLENDED COMPOUND AND ALTERNATING EXERCISES. (See movements under Definitions and Explanations in Appendix.)

The following illustrates, in a condensed form, the possibilities of combining different arm movements with any one leg movement. Each arm movement, combined with a leg movement, constitutes an exercise. It is not to be interpreted that these exercises are taken serially.

The possibilities for making similar combinations are limited only by the ingenuity of the teacher.

1. Jump between stride standing and standing with:
    (a) Arm raising sideways.
    (b) Hand clapping over head.
    (c) (Bend standing) Single and double arm stretching sideways and downward.
    (d) Double, single, and alternate arm stretching upward, sideways, forward and downward.
    (e) (Bend standing) Single and double arm stretching sideways and downward.
    (f) Arm swinging forward and sideways.

(g) Arm swinging forward and sideways and circling.

(h) Arm flinging between cross and fly.

(i) Alternate and double arm flinging (forward upward) between drag and stretch.

(j) Arm swinging between reach, fold, arm side, and in reverse order.

(k) Arm placing sideways, bending, stretching upward, placing sideways, bending, stretching forward, bending, stretching downward.

2. Heel raising and knee bending with:

(a) Alternate or double arm swinging forward—backward.

(b) Arm swinging forward and sideways.

(c) Arm swinging forward and sideways and circling.

(d) (Bend standing) Arm stretching upward, sideways, forward, and downward.

(e) Double, single and alternate arm stretching upward, sideways, forward, and downward.

(f) Arm swinging forward and sideways (holding one arm one count every 4th count).

(g) Arm flinging between cross and fly.

(h) Arm flinging between fold and arm side.

(i) Alternate and double arm flinging (forward-upward) between drag and stretch.

(j) Arm swinging between reach, fold, arm side, and in reverse order.

3. Heel raising and knee bending and alternate knee lifting with:

  All (a—j) under No. 2.

  Combination of (j) and exercise (23) page 104.

4. Quick deep knee bending (from toe standing) with:

  (a), (b), (d), (g), (i), (j), under No. 2.

5. Two hops with alternate leg flinging sideways with:

  (a) (Bend standing) Arm stretching sideways (may be alternate and opposite).

  (b) (Bend standing) Arm stretching upward (may be alternate and opposite).

  (c) Arm stretching upward and sideways.

  (d) Left (right) arm stretching sideways and right (left) arm stretching upward.

  (e) Alternate arm swinging sideways-upward to top of head.

  (f) Double, single and alternate arm stretching upward, sideways, forward and downward.

  (g) Arm swinging forward and sideways (holding one arm one count every 4th count).

  (h) Arm flinging between cross and fly.

  (i) Arm flinging between reach, fold, arm side, and in reverse order.

6. Back lying alternate knee lifting (and stretching upward) with:

  (a) Arm bending and stretching upward.

(b) Arm bending and stretching sideways.

(c) Arm bending and stretching upward, sideways, forward, and downward.

(d) Arm swinging between reach, fold, arm side, and in reverse order.

(e) Opposite and double arm bending and stretching in all directions.

7. Two hops with alternate leg flinging sideways with alternate arm swinging sideways, upward to top of head.

8. Three or four hops with alternate leg swinging in circle with opposite arm swinging sideways-upward to top of head.

9. Four hops with alternate toe touching sideways and knee lifting and toe touching forward and knee lifting and a quick deep knee bending followed by a quarter turn left or right.

(a) Double, single and alternate arm stretching.

(b) Double, single and alternate arm placing between reach, fold and arm side.

10. Jump and alternate heel touching forward and toe touching in place with:

(a) Low hand clapping in front of body.

(b) Many other arm movements.

The following exercises are analyzed according to movement and count.

11. Back lying, lift left knee and raise both arms vertically forward (palms facing knee) .... 1 count

Bend ankle and wrist (toward each other) .... 1 count

Extend ankle and wrists (away from each other) .... 1 count

Bend ankle and wrists.............. 1 count

Relax wrists and ankle............. 1 count

Replace arms and leg.............. 1 count

Raise arms and right knee ready to repeat .... 1 count

_____

7 counts

12. Erect standing—walk forward 4 steps with arm swinging forward and sideways .... 4 counts

Hold arms in reach position as left knee is lifted.................... 1 count

Bend ankle and wrists toward each other .... 1 count

Stretch ankle and bend wrists away from each other................ 1 count

Walk backward 4 steps swinging arms sideways and forward............ 4 counts

Hold arms sideways and (in this position) repeat the bending and stretching of ankle and wrists.......... 3 counts

_____

14 counts

For variation—One arm may be raised forward as the other is raised sideways, before the bending and stretching of ankle and wrists.

13. Two hops with alternate leg flinging
sideways with double arm swinging
sideways .... 4 counts
Two hops with alternate knee lifting
with arm swinging forward and sideways .... 4 counts

    _____

    8 counts

14. Jump from squat sitting to stride
standing and standing with hand clapping over head and arm bending and
stretching.

    Jump to squat sitting, hands on thighs. 1 count
    Jump to stride standing with hand
        clapping over head............. 1 count
    Jump to standing with arms at side.. 1 count
    Jump in place bending arms (with
        hands at shoulders).............. 1 count
    Jump in place stretching arms side-
        ways .... 1 count

    _____

    5 counts

    For variation—A quarter turn left
    (right) may be made with the change
    from the first to the second count.

15. Alternate arm swinging (one forward,
one backward) with alternate heel
raising .... 4 counts
Alternate arm circling (one forward,
one backward) .... 4 counts

    _____

    8 counts

3, 5 or 7 steps forward and backward may be combined with No. 15.

16. Bend standing hop with alternate toe touching sideways and turning with toe touching forward and quick deep knee bending with arm stretching sideways and forward.

Hop with left toe touching sideways with arm stretching sideways and arm bending .... 2 counts
Turn left with hop and alternate toe touching forward with arm stretching forward and arm bending.... 2 counts
Quick deep knee bending with hands supported on thighs.............. 2 counts
_____
6 counts

17. Hop with alternate toe touching sideways and foot lifting backward (knee bent).

Hop with left toe touching sideways.. 1 count
Hop changing to toe touching right.. 1 count
Hop on right foot raising left leg backward .... 1 count
_____
3 counts

Repeat all starting right

Various arm movements may be combined with No. 17.

18. Hop with alternate heel and toe touching forward and opposite leg lifting backward (knee bent).

Hop with left heel touching forward. 1 count
Hop with left toe touching forward... 1 count
Hop on left foot raising right leg backward (knee slightly bent)........ 1 count

_____

3 counts

Repeat same starting with right

Various arm movements may be combined with No. 18

19. Bend standing hop with alternate toe touching sideways and forward and ¼ turns with arm stretching sideways and forward followed by deep knee bending.

Bend standing hop with alternate toe touching sideways with arm stretching sideways and bending........ 2 counts
Quarter turn left and alternate toe touching forward with arm stretching forward and bending......... 2 counts
Jump to deep knee bending with hands on thighs .... 2 counts

_____

6 counts

The following illustrate the use that may be made of various arm movements combined with a trunk and a leg movement.

20. Grasp hook sitting (hands on feet) alternate and double leg stretching.

> Note: After the double leg stretching the arms may be placed sideways on level of shoulders as the back is stretched.
>
> See illustration 20
>
> Page 160

21. Grasp half hook lying head bending forward alternating with chest lifting.

    Combination of exercises 90 and 102.

22. Arm side back lying head and alternate knee lifting alternating with chest lifting with arm and leg raising.

The following exercises are analyzed according to movement and count.

23. Stride standing trunk bending downward (striking floor) and:

    (a) Arm flinging between drag and stretch.

    Trunk bending downward hands striking floor .... 1 count
    Trunk raising forward to angle standing while arms are swung backward to drag position................. 1 count
    Trunk raising to erect standing and bending downward again as the arms are swung forcefully upward and backward .... 1 count
    _____
    3 counts

(b) Arm flinging between cross and fly.

(c) Arm flinging between fold and side arm.

24. Hand squat sitting knee stretching with trunk springing and arm flinging between cross and fly.

Knee stretching with trunk springing. 1 count
Angle standing arm flinging between
   cross and fly..................... 1 count
Trunk springing .... 1 count
Return to position................ 1 count

                                4 counts

25. Hand squat sitting double leg stretching backward with a jump back to
   squat sitting .... 2 counts
Knee stretching with trunk springing 1 count
Forward stretching of trunk with arm
   flinging between cross and fly...... 1 count
Trunk springing .... 1 count
Knee bending with hands on floor.... 1 count

                                6 counts

26. Heel raising with slow arm stretching and heel sinking with trunk bending downward followed by trunk raising and alternate high knee lifting and stretching with alternate (same or opposite) slow arm stretching.

Heel raising with slow arm stretching (through bend) over head...... 2 counts
Heel sinking with arm lowering backward, sideways-downward .... 2 counts
Slow trunk bending downward to
grasp ankles and arm bending..... 4 counts
Trunk raising .... 2 counts
Left high knee lifting and stretching
and sinking with slow right arm
stretching over head............. 3 counts
Right high knee lifting and stretching and sinking with slow left arm
stretching over head............. 3 counts

—————————

16 counts

27. Head bending forward with alternate
knee lifting (hands grasping knees)
and trunk bending downward (to
grasp ankles) with arm bending followed by trunk raising with chest
lifting and low hand turning.

Head bending forward with left knee
lifting (hands grasping knees).... 2 counts
Head bending forward with right
knee lifting (hands grasping knees) 2 counts
Trunk bending downward to grasp
ankles with arm bending.......... 2 counts
Trunk raising .... 2 counts
Chest lifting with low hand turning
or arm stretching (through bend)
overhead and sideways-downward.. 2 counts

—————————

10 counts

28. Knee standing arm swinging forward and sideways with alternate leg stretching sideways and side bending (4 times) followed by (half knee standing) arm swinging forward and sideways with trunk bending forward (straightening forward knee).

Knee standing arm swinging forward .... 1 count

Arm swinging sideways with leg stretching sideways and arm swing forward and to "S" standing...... 3 counts

"S" ½ knee stride standing side bending (4 times).................... 4 counts
_____
8 counts

Arm swinging outward-downward and forward with leg replacing....... 1 count

Repeat counts 2–8 taken to opposite side .... 7 counts
_____
8 counts

(Exercise may be terminated and repeated here or the following may be added.)

Half knee standing (left or right leg forward) arm swinging forward... 1 count

Arm swinging sideways-upward overhead with downward bending of trunk (straightening forward knee) 3 counts

Trunk springing (4 times)......... 4 counts
_____
8 counts

Trunk raising with arm swinging sideways and forward with leg changing 4 counts
Repeat on opposite side............. 4 counts

_____

8 counts

_____

16 counts

29. Bend standing hop with alternate toe
touching sideways and forward and
deep knee bending followed by a
jump to stride (with trunk bent forward) and arm flinging between
drag and stretch and deep knee bending. (Rhythm uneven.)

Bend standing hop with alternate toe
touching sideways and forward with
alternate (opposite) arm stretching
sideways and forward............ 4 counts
Jump to deep knee bending......... 2 counts
Jump to stride angle standing with
arm flinging between drag and
stretch. (Repeat 4 times)......... 8 counts
Jump to deep knee bending......... 2 counts

_____

16 counts

30. Hand squat sitting hop with alternate
leg stretching sideways .... 5 counts
Double leg stretching backward (2
times) .... 4 counts

B. COMBINATIONS

A combination is a group of three or more exercises which (on separate signal) permit an easy transition from one to another, and are so arranged that different regions are included and various effects attained.

The following are only a few suggestions of possible combinations.

1. Hop between stride and standing with hand clapping overhead.
2. Stride angle standing arm flinging between drag and stretch.
3. Hand squat sitting alternate leg stretching sideways or knee stretching.

1. Arm swinging forward and sideways with alternate foot placing sideways.
2. Grasp bow standing arm bending and trunk raising with chest lifting.
3. Stride angle standing arm flinging between drag and stretch.

1. Back lying alternate knee bending and stretching with help of hands.
2. Back lying head and alternate knee bending upward and chest lifting.
3. Alternate knee bending and stretching with arm movements.
4. Arm side back lying slow trunk bending forward to grasp ankles.

1. Long sitting arm flinging between cross and fly and trunk springing.
2. Grasp hook sitting (hands on knees) chest lifting.

3. Grasp hook sitting (hands on feet) alternate and double leg stretching.

1. Stride standing single arm circling.
2. Top standing alternate knee bending and stretching and pushing off.
3. Half wing stride standing trunk twisting with single arm flinging.
4. Hop between stride standing and standing with hand clapping over head.

1. Hop between stride standing and standing with hand clapping over head.
2. Stride standing arm flinging between cross and fly.
3. Neck stride bow standing trunk springing.
4. Hand squat sitting knee stretching with trunk springing.

1. Stride standing arm flinging between cross and fly with heel raising.
2. Half wing stride standing trunk twisting with single arm flinging.
3. Half grasp stride bow standing trunk springing.

1. Hand knee standing trunk twisting with single arm flinging.
2. Hand knee standing arm bending and knee stretching.
3. Back clasp knee bow sitting chest lifting (or stretching).

1. Arm swinging forward and sideways with alternate foot placing sideways.

2. "S" stride standing side bending of trunk with alternate toe touching sideways.
3. Neck stride bow standing trunk springing and back stretching.

1. Leg flinging forward and backward with hand clapping over head.
2. Trunk bending downward to grasp ankles with arm bending followed by trunk raising with chest lifting.
3. Half wing stride standing trunk twisting with single arm flinging.

1. Back lying trunk bending forward.
2. Back lying alternate knee bending and stretching with help of hands.
3. Arm side back lying chest lifting alternating with head and alternate knee lifting.

1. Jump with alternate knee lifting and opposite arm swinging forward.
2. Stride standing arm flinging between cross and fly.
3. Half grasp stride bow standing trunk springing.

1. Trunk bending downward to grasp ankles with arm bending (or trunk springing).
2. Arm flinging from cross to fly with heel raising and knee bending and single knee lifting.
3. Wing standing hop with alternate toe touching sideways and forward.

1. Back lying trunk bending forward to slap floor.
2. Long sitting leg lifting with help.
3. Hurdle sitting trunk bending forward.

4. Hand knee standing trunk twisting with **arm** flinging.

1. Jump in place.
2. Heel raising and knee bending with arm flinging between cross and fly.
3. Hand squat sitting knee stretching with trunk springing and arm flinging between cross and fly.

1. Half wing stride standing trunk twisting with arm flinging.
2. Half grasp stride bow standing trunk springing changing with twist.
3. Hand half squat stride standing alternate knee stretching and bending.
4. "S" stride standing side bending with opposite knee bending.

C. SERIES—

A series is a succession of movements repeated in a given order upon an initial signal.

Long and involved series of this type are not advocated for use in America except in situations where learned "drills" are still in use. Countless exercises of this nature could be invented, if desired, and executed in response to a single initial signal, but to accurately perform these presupposes a great deal of learning and drilling, and after this has been accomplished there is little value in it except for exhibition purposes. For America, at least, it is felt advisable that this type of work should be greatly minimized, and it is given here merely as an example of the possibilities of variation.

The complexity and dissimilarity of these movements make them difficult to name and a count for each element has therefore been given.

1. Jump to stride standing with hand
   clapping over head.............. 1 count
   Jump to position................ 1 count
   Jump in place .... 1 count
   Jump to stride standing with arm rais-
   ing sideways .... 1 count
   Jump to position .... 1 count
   Jump in place .... 1 count
   Jump to stride standing with arm rais-
   ing sideways .... 1 count
   Jump to position................ 1 count
   Jump in place .... 1 count
   Jump to stride standing with arm rais-
   ing sideways .... 1 count
   Jump to position................ 1 count
   Jump to half knee bending hands on
   hips .... 1 count
   Knee stretching with heel raising with
   arm bending .... 1 count
   Heel sinking with arm stretching over-
   head .... 1 count
   Heel raising with arm bending...... 1 count
   Knee bending with arm stretching side-
   ways .... 1 count
   Knee stretching with heel raising with
   arm bending .... 1 count
   Heel sinking with arm stretching forward .... 1 count
   Heel raising with arm bending...... 1 count
   Knee bending with arm stretching
   downward .... 1 count
   (to start swing outward-upward to
   repeat exercise)

   _____

   20 counts

2. Arm swinging forward and sideways
    and arm circling with heel raising
    and easy knee bending .... 4 counts
   Arm swinging forward and sideways
    with foot placing sideways and arm
    circling and swinging forward and
    sideways to "S" stride standing... 4 counts
   "S" stride standing side bending with
    opposite knee bending (4 bendings). 4 counts
   Arm swinging outward-downward with
    foot replacing and arm swinging for-
    ward with heel raising and knee
    bending with arm swinging sideways
    and circling .... 4 counts
                                   _____
                                   ·16 counts
   Repeat last 12 counts taken to the op-
    posite side ....12 counts
                                   _____
                                   28 counts
   (Exercise may be terminated and re-
    peated here, or the following may be
    added.)

Arm swinging forward and sideways
and arm circling with heel raising
and easy knee bending .... 4 counts

Arm swinging forward and sideways
with foot placing and with trunk
twisting obliquely forward and arm
circling and arm swinging forward
and sideways .... 4 counts

Trunk springing (4 times) .... 4 counts

Arm swinging backward, forward, sideways with trunk raising and foot replacing with arm swinging sideways
and circling with heel raising ..... 4 counts

Repeat last 12 counts taken to the opposite side ....12 counts

—————————

28 counts

CHAPTER X

SELF-TESTING ACTIVITIES ON APPARATUS AND MATS.
JUMPING, VAULTING AND AGILITY EXERCISES, IN-
CLUDING A FEW SUSPENSION EXERCISES

The exercises listed in this section may supplement a gymnastic lesson or may be used for an entire class period.

This form of activity is not necessarily used to train the muscles or to give the joints more mobility, but to increase and test the power to control and co-ordinate acquired flexibility and strength. The jumps, deep springs, and light landings involved in many of the floor exercises, are a contributing factor in the execution of the vaults and jumps.

Although not necessary, it is advisable to begin with simple jumps, using multiple apparatus, and progress to the more difficult exercises as the proficiency of the class increases.

The class may be in rank formation so that as many as possible start on the same signal and perform the same jump.

By this arrangement, individual criticisms and admonitions are possible. It is also a help to the more timid, less agile members, for *turns* come often and they do not feel so self-conscious.

This multiple or mass organization of apparatus is used by Mr. Bukh to supplement a gymnastic lesson. The work is easily adapted to squad organization with different apparatus activities in each squad.

116

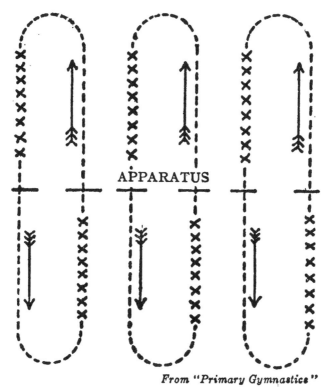

APPARATUS

From "Primary Gymnastics"

Fɪɢ. I.—Used in Denmark.

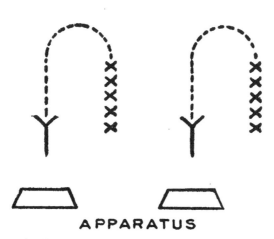

APPARATUS

Fɪɢ. II.—Used in America, two or more pieces of apparatus **may** be used.

A. JUMPING AND VAULTING

(See illustration 1, page 162.)

As this book is intended for trained teachers of physical education, who are entirely familiar with most of the self-testing activities on the floor and apparatus that are listed in "Grundgymnastik," the translators feel it necessary to describe in detail only those vaults and jumps which are unusual or unique in their agility content, and which might be used to good advantage in apparatus progression.

In the execution of these activities, there should be no tension or stiffness and they should be performed easily and in 'good form,' omitting all exaggerated, unnecessary formality in the 'finish' and on the landings.

All jumps and vaults are preceded by light runs and 'take offs,' and an exercise is terminated by a light deep knee spring on the landing.

1. *Preliminary jump over low apparatus* (Box 14 inches in height)

   May be executed over a rope, bench, low boom or (top) section of the box, and may be taken with or without a definite number of running steps. This should be practiced with the chest lifted,—head held high,—and with a double as well as a single foot 'take off.'

2. *Preliminary jump with double or single foot 'take off' on low apparatus*

   The same 'take off' as for the preceding jump, except that a landing is made on the top of the apparatus, followed by immediate dismount from the box, chest lifted, head held high. On the dismount, the arms may be swung sideways or forward-upward.

3. *Running jump*

May be performed over the same apparatus, from a single foot 'take off,' landing on far side of apparatus on the opposite foot, and continuing the run as a hurdle is incorporated in a run. The arms may be raised diagonally forward upward as the leap over the apparatus is made.

4. *Running jump with turns left and right*

This jump is the same as No. 3 except that a complete turn is made in the air, either left or right, as directed. On the left foot 'take off,' a left turn is made and the landing is made on the right foot. The run is continued without a pause as in No. 3.

5. *Kneeling mount, "courage" vault dismount*

(See illustration 2, page 162.)

Apparatus:	Box—horse—buck.
Approach:	Running
Take off:	Double
Execution:	Hands placed quickly on apparatus and at same time knees are flexed and brought between the hands so as to finish in a kneeling position.
Dismount:	As arms are swung forcefully forward a spring from the knees is made, bringing the knees to the chest as a deep knee spring landing is made on the floor, in front of the apparatus.

6. *Standing mount*

(See illustration 2, page 162.)

Apparatus:	Same as for No. 5.
Approach:	Running.
Take off:	Double.
Execution:	Hands are placed quickly on the apparatus and pushed off again as the feet, with knees quickly flexed, are brought up to a standing position on the apparatus.
Dismount:	Backward—or immediately forward — or arms may be swung forward and sideways with heel raising and knee bending preceding the jump dismount.
Assistance on landing:	A person may receive by grasping the hands of the performer and stepping backward, each executing a deep knee spring on the landing.

7. *Knee chest vault*

Apparatus: (crosswise)	. Boom, saddle-boom, box, horse, buck.
Approach:	Running.
Take off:	Double.
Execution:	Hands placed on and parallel to long way of the apparatus. Body is swung

to one side, up and over apparatus, knees and hip joints fully flexed. Hips are held high with weight of body over straight arms.

Landing: Facing box or a 90° to 180° turn.

8. *Rear vault*

Apparatus: Box, horse, buck.
a. (lengthwise)
Approach: Straight running.
Take off: Double, one side of center of apparatus.
Execution: Both hands placed on and parallel to long way of apparatus, left (right) hand pushes off and the back is turned toward the apparatus at the same time the legs are swung forward-upward to an angle of 45°. Legs straight and together.
Landing: Left (right) side against apparatus—left (right) hand grasping apparatus while other hand remains at side.
b. (crosswise)
Approach: Straight running, then slightly to side (L or R) just within a few steps

of place where "take off"
is made.

Take off: Double.
Execution: Same.
Landing: Same.

9. *Oblique vault*

Apparatus: Box, horse, buck.

10. *Straddle vault*

Apparatus: Buck: (lengthwise or crosswise).

11. *Squat vault*

Apparatus: Buck, side or long-horse,
saddle-boom, box.

12. *High jump*

Apparatus: Over high a p p a r a t u s
(men's exercise).
Horse, box or buck (lengthwise or crosswise).

13. *"Thief" vault*

Apparatus: Side horse, buck (crosswise), box.

Approach: Long run, gaining momentum.

Take off: Single foot.

Execution: This vault begins as a high
jump, but after the feet
and legs have passed over
the apparatus the hands

reach back, grasp the pommels on apparatus, and with a strong push off, give the body the necessary lift to clear the apparatus. It is important that the feet swing high and precede the body, (which leans backward), as the vault is made.

Landing: Deep knee spring.

Assistance: It is helpful, for girls at least, to have two people receive on the far side and facing the apparatus, ready to grasp the performer's arms as the dismount is made.

B. SUSPENSION EXERCISES ON APPARATUS

In a gymnasium where vertical ropes are arranged in suitable relation to the boom, the following very interesting agility exercises may be given.

1. *Grasp standing forward swing to knee hanging position on boom*

(See illustration 3, page 163.)

Apparatus: Vertical ropes; boom chest high.

Approach: Short run.

Take off: Single, as jump to a bent arm position is made.

Execution: As body is lifted and swung forward, legs are raised, k n e e s straight (right angle at hip), and then knees are hooked over the boom. The body is then lowered backward slowly by sliding hands down the ropes. The ropes are set free as the hands are placed on the floor. In this position, the body s h o u l d be supported easily on the hands while hanging from the knees. (It is important that the abdominal muscles be contracted.)

Dismount: Made by lifting the feet and legs from the boom and flexing the hips (and later the knees), landing on the feet in a hand squat position.

Variation: Later the boom may be raised and a dismount made on the back or shoulders (men) of a p e r s o n kneeling (or standing (men) on hands and knees.

Assistance: Far or near side.
It is important and advisable to have assistance in

this activity, even on the low boom. One hand is placed on the feet of the performer which are on the far side of the boom. As the dismount is made, the opposite hand is placed on the abdomen, and the hand which has supported the feet is placed on the lower back to help in the control of the hips.

2. *Grasp standing forward swing to standing position on the boom*

(See illustration 4, page 163.)

Apparatus:	Vertical ropes; boom—between level of chest and knee (with flat edge upward).
Approach: Take off:	} Same as for No. 1.
Execution:	As body is swung forward, a drop is made on to the boom. An erect standing position must be maintained for a few moments after the ropes are set free or until a signal for dismount is given.
Dismount:	Deep spring forward.

3. *Grasp standing forward swing to sitting position on boom*

(See illustration 5, page 164.)

Apparatus: Vertical ropes; boom shoulder height.

Approach: }
Take off: } Same as for No. 1.

Execution: The legs are swung upward (knees straight) over the boom (right angle in hip joints). The body drops to a sitting position on the boom as the ropes are set free. The hands immediately grasp the boom (fingers forward, thumbs back).

Dismount: a. The legs are d r a w n slightly back and then swung quickly forward, and a push off with the hands is given as the deep-spring dismount is made.

b. The performer s l i d e s forward into a back-rest position on boom (elbows straight). A backward circle is made to inverted hanging position. The hips and knees are then flexed, and dismount is made.

(See illustration 6 b, page 164.)

4. *Forward circle to front rest*

(See illustration 6 a, page 164.)

Side riding rest with arm swinging forward and sideways may be taken.

5. *Fall hanging arm bending*

(See illustration 7, page 165.)

Apparatus: Boom; vertical ropes; incline low ladder (hip height).

Position: a. Over grasp (e l b o w s straight), body extended f o r w a r d (resting on heels) or,

b. Assisted by helper who holds performer's feet as he would the handles of a wheelbarrow, and pushes slightly forward.

Execution: Arms bent at elbows, chest forward, chin in, straight line from top of head to heels.

May also be taken from long-sitting position with trunk raising and arm bending.

6. *Hanging arm bending*

(See illustration 8, page 165.)

Apparatus: Boom, horizontal bar, ladder, vertical ropes, or **rings** (over head, high).

Position:	Over grasp.
Execution:	Elbows must be forced backward as arms are bent, head back and chin held in. Alternate or double knee bending may be executed during the arm bending.
Assistance:	May be given by putting a hand at the back of the performer's head.

7. *Hanging—shoulder stretching*

(See illustration 9, page 165.)

Apparatus:	Double-boom, (second bar at height of shoulder blades.)
Execution:	a. H a n g i n g, over-grasp with straight arms.
	b. May be assisted by helper who holds performer's feet as he would hold the handles of a wheelbarrow.
Execution:	a. The body is swung easily and gently forward and backward.
	b. The helper gently pushes the performer's b o d y against the lower bar, putting a strong stretch on the chest muscles.

C. SELF-TESTING OR AGILITY ACTIVITIES ON THE MAT

BIBLIOGRAPHY:

"Health by Stunts," *P*earl and Brown—MacMillan & Co.

"*P*rimary Gymnastics," Niels Bukh—Methuen & Co., England.

"Agility exercises are, in Denmark, the most popular of all exercises for men and boys. They develop strength, nimbleness and skill. They are most enjoyable. There is just that slight touch of danger in some of them which makes them appeal to healthy boys. Finally, they re-quire very little or no apparatus, as they may be performed on a lawn or in a field. They form part of nearly all schemes of work for boys in Danish schools." "*P*rimary Gymnastics," page 23.

1. Forward roll.
2. Hand stand—assisted or unassisted.
3. Head stand—illustration 10, page 166.
4. Cartwheel.
5. Backward roll.
6. Backward roll to head stand.
7. Backward roll to hand stand.[1]
8. Hand spring (double foot take off).[2]

> Note: can be taken also on low box, horse, buck, or box—crosswise.

9. Head spring (double foot take off).[3]
10. Hand spring (single foot take off) illustration 11, page 166.

[1] Boys and men.
[2] Boys and men.
[3] Boys and men.

Like hand stand, but speed so great that performer passes through the hand stand position and lands on his feet. Arms are not kept fully stretched—a slight give in elbows—with a strong push off. May be taken from a standing position or with a short run, in which case the run finishes with a little hop while the foot that is to be used for the take off is brought forward.

11. "Flip-flap" (double foot take off).

After a run and a strong take off, the performer jumps forward-upward in a curve. The hip joints may be slightly bent, or stretched. He lands on his hands, the arms yield slightly and immediately push off so as to help in swinging the body around. The landing is taken as No. 8.

For beginners it is an advantage to place the hands on a higher level than the take off and the landing. For this, two or three mats may be piled on top of each other. There is an element of danger here, so great care should be taken in receiving. The preceding stunts may be combined in various ways. In the following, examples are given of combinations that may be taken according to the class arrangeme t shown in the illustration on page 166.

12. Hand spring—head spring.
13. Hand spring—flip-flap.
14. Two head springs in succession.
15. Head spring, jump about—backward roll with a jump about.
16. Walking on hands.

CHAPTER V

A. ARM POSITIONS

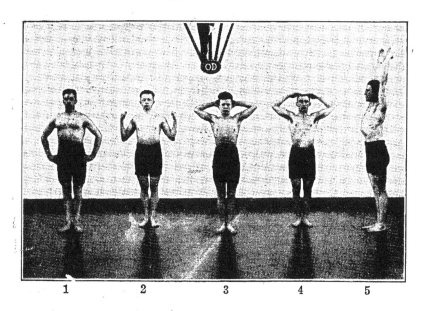

1 2 3 4 5

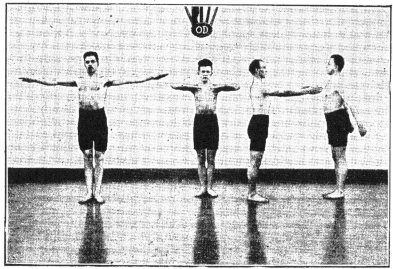

6 7 8 9

NOTE. The illustrations of Starting Positions and Exercises are numbered to correspond to the numbers given the exercises in the respective chapters.

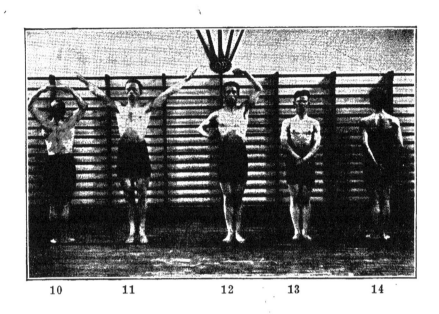

10   11   12   13   14

B. LEG POSITIONS

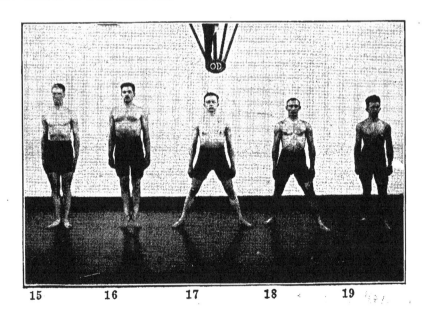

15   16   17   18   19

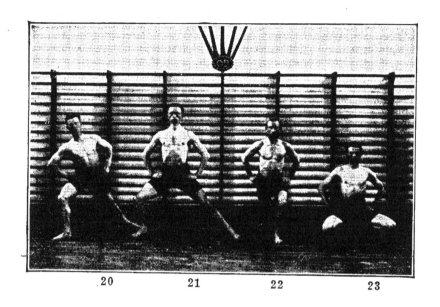

20   21   22   23

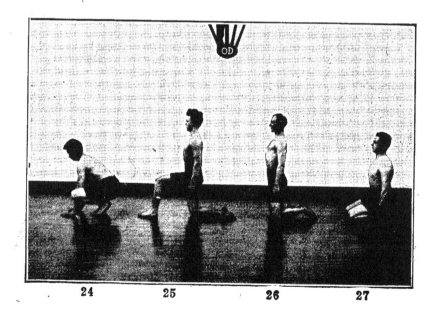

24   25   26   27

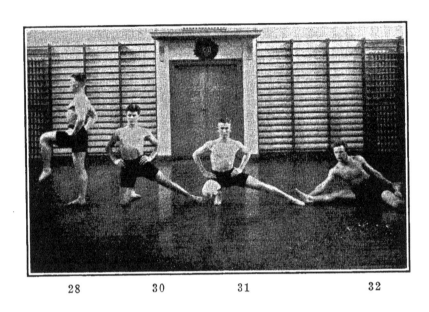

28   30   31   32

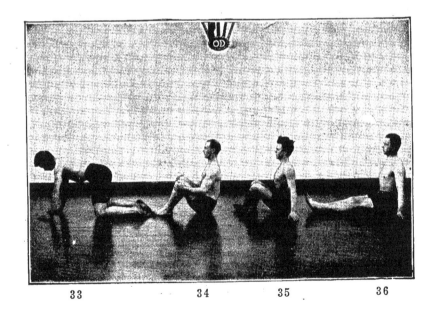

33   34   35   36

C. TRUNK POSITIONS

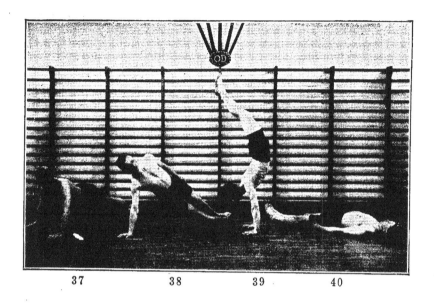

37 38 39 40

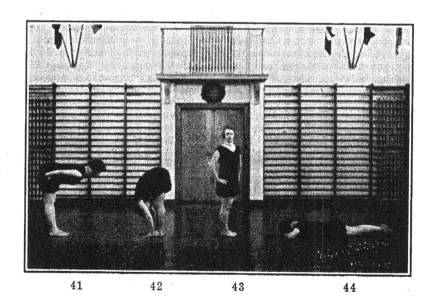

41 42 43 44

D. BAR STALL POSITIONS

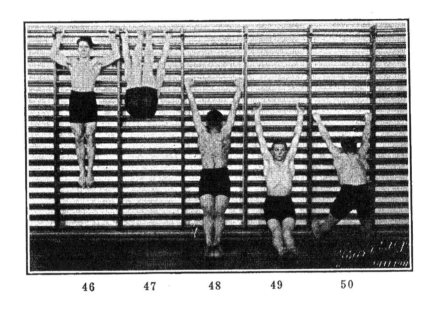

46   47   48   49   50

CHAPTER VI

Exercises for Flexibility

A. LEGS AND HIP JOINTS

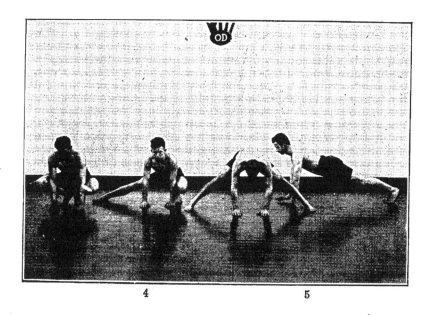

4 5

B. LEGS, HIP JOINTS AND LOWER BACK

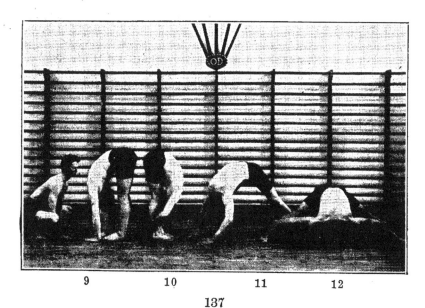

9 10 11 12

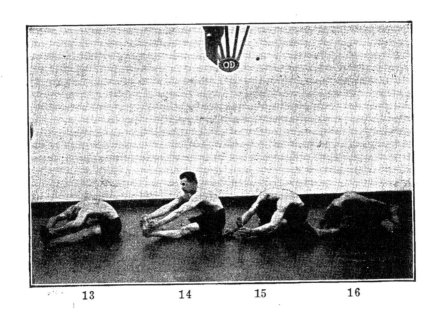

13   14   15   16

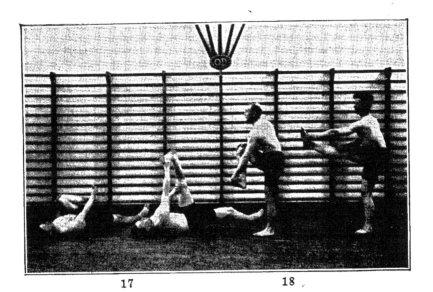

17   18

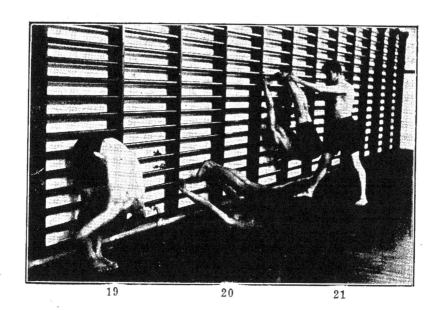

19   20   21

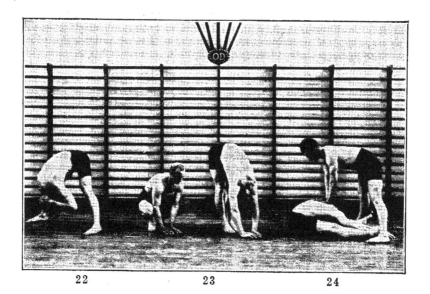

22   23   24

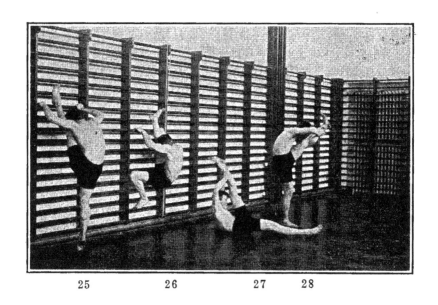

25 26 27 28

C. ARMS AND SHOULDER GIRDLE

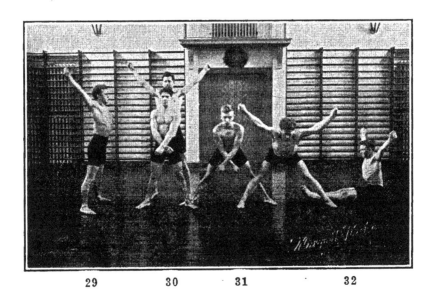

29 30 31 32

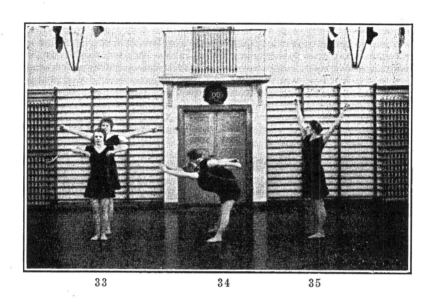

33   34   35

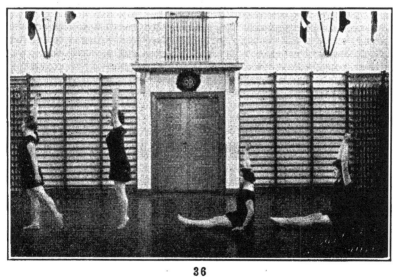

36

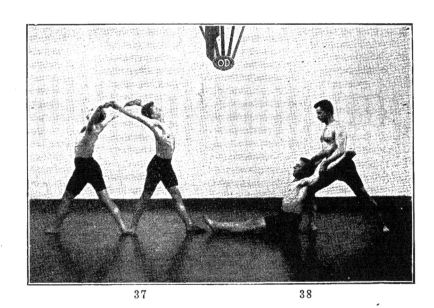

37   38

D. NECK AND UPPER BACK

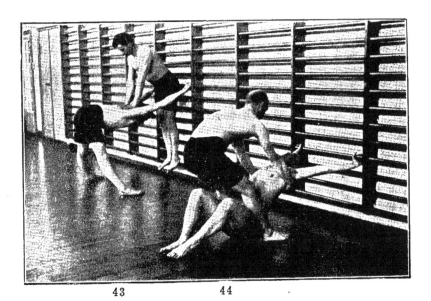

43   44

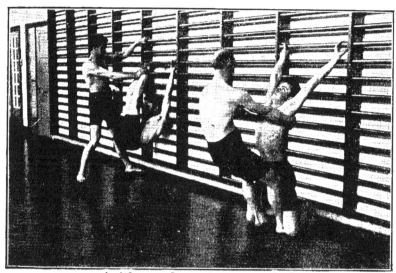

(with supplementary exercise)

45

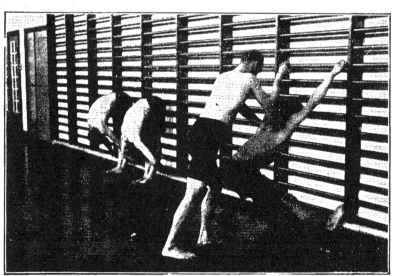

(with supplementary exercise)

46

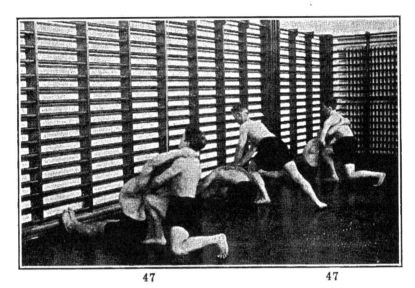

47   47

neck grasp   waist grasp

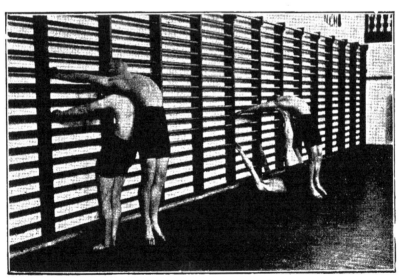

48   49

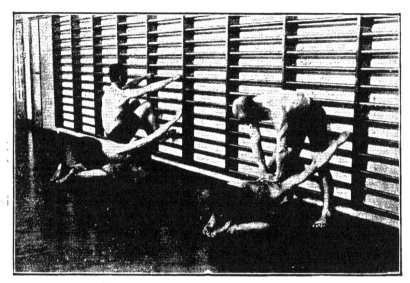

50

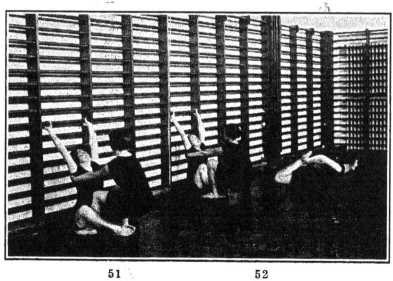

51   52

E. LATERAL TRUNK

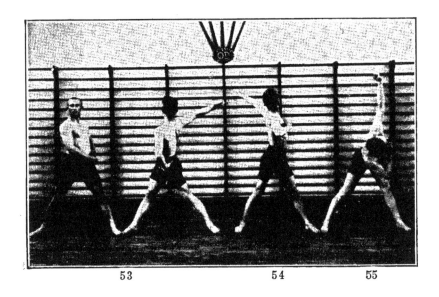

53   54   55

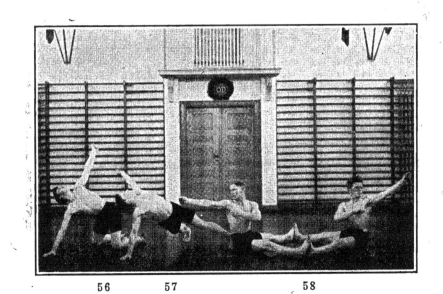

56   57   58

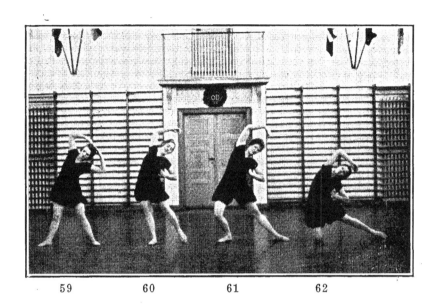

59   60   61   62

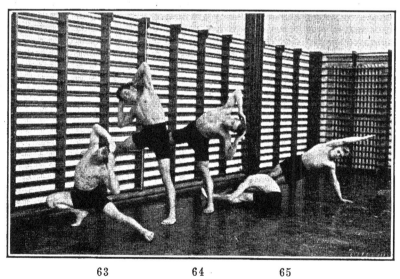

63   64   65

CHAPTER VII

Exercises for Strength

A. LEGS

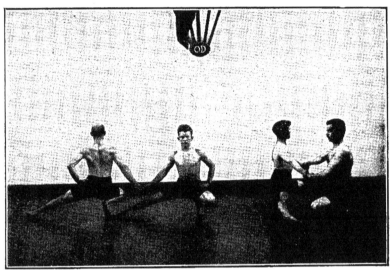

68

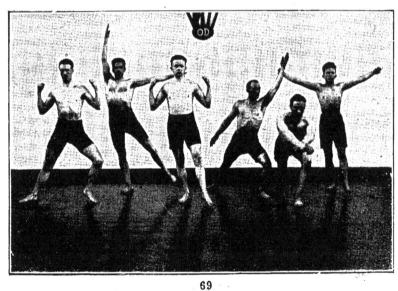

69

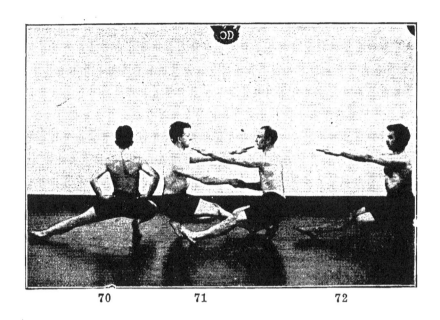

70   71   72

B. ARMS AND SHOULDER GIRDLE

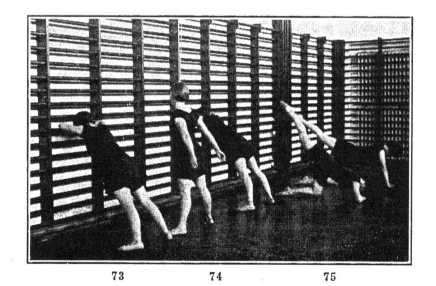

73   74   75

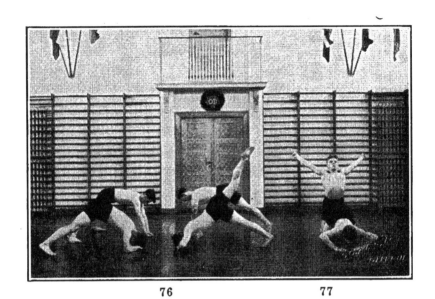

76   77

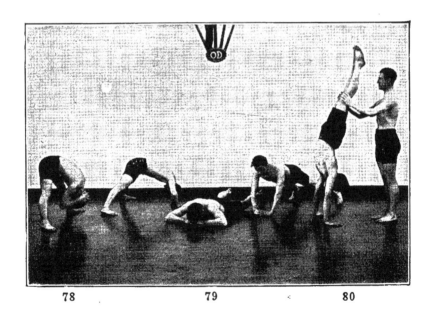

78   79   80

C. ARMS AND BACK

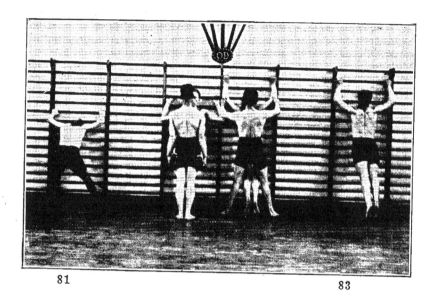

81   83

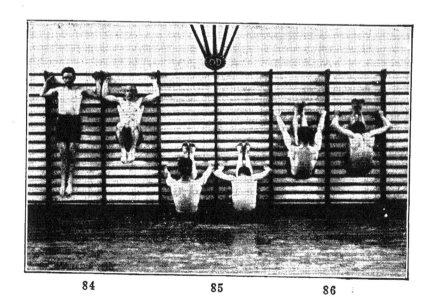

84   85   86

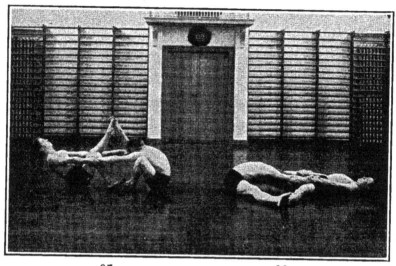

87   88

D. NECK AND BACK

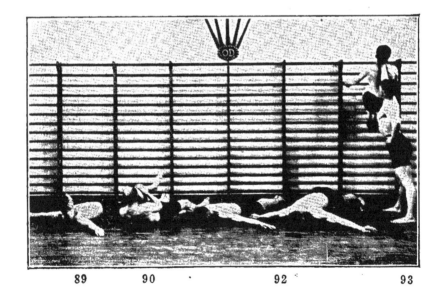

89   90   92   93

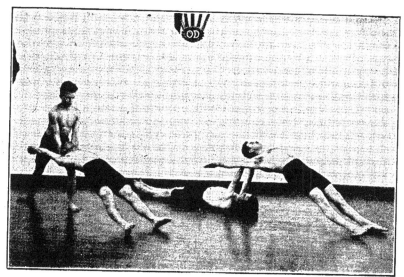

94

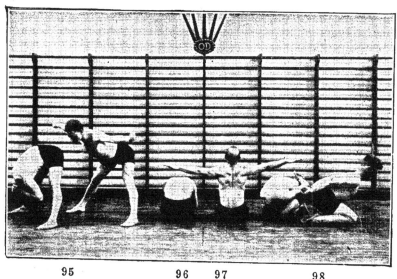

95   96   97   98

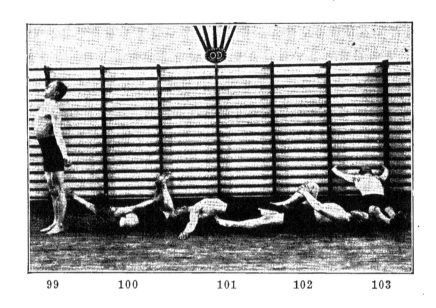

99   100   101   102   103

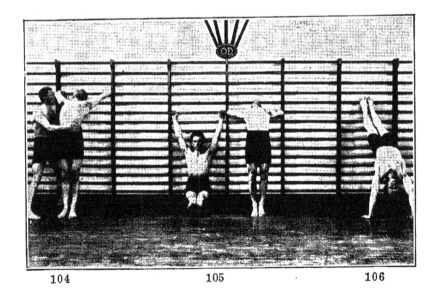

104   105   106

E. ABDOMEN

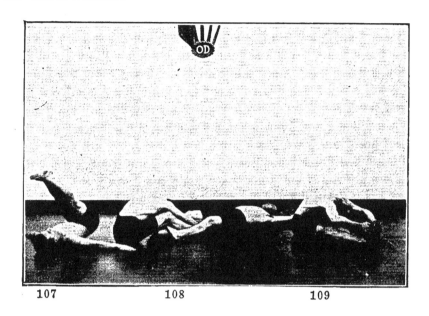

107   108   109

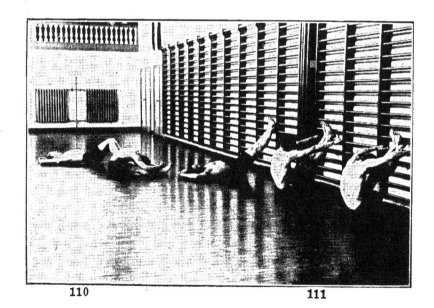

110   111

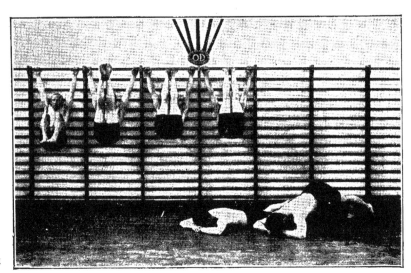

112   113

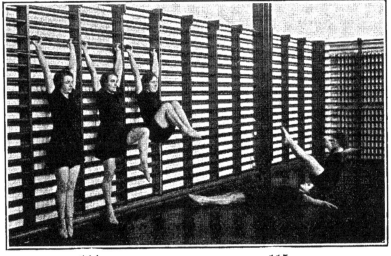

114   115

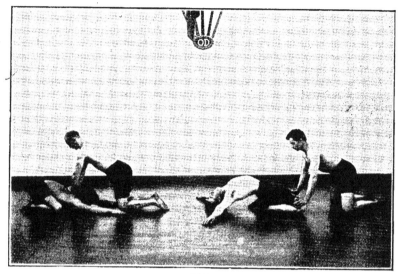

116

F. LATERAL TRUNK

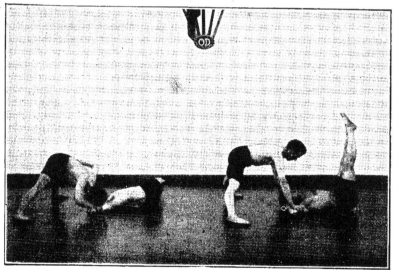

118

CHAPTER VIII

EXERCISES FOR CO-ORDINATION

A. LEGS

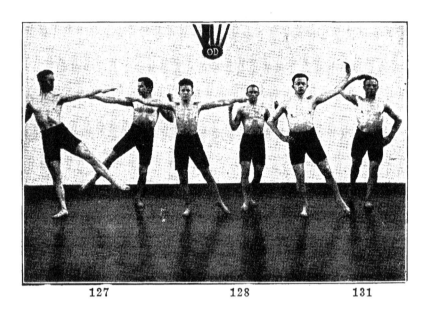

127   128   131

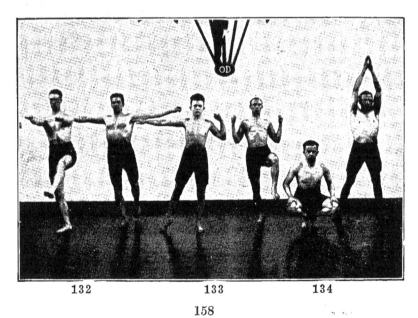

132   133   134

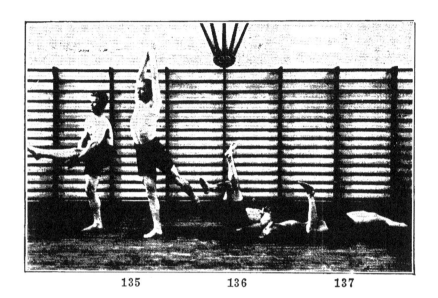

135   136   137

CHAPTER IX

COMBINED EXERCISES

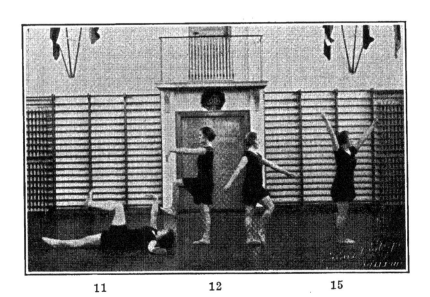

11   12   15

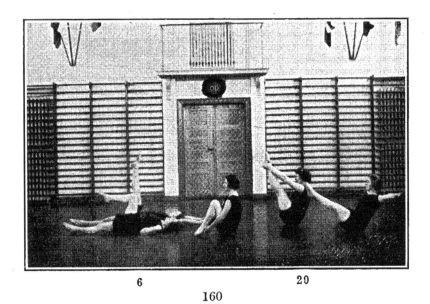

6   20

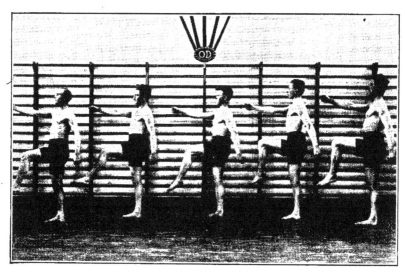

FIRM WALK

See Chapter III.

CHAPTER X

SELF-TESTING ACTIVITIES ON APPARATUS AND MATS

A. JUMPING AND VAULTING

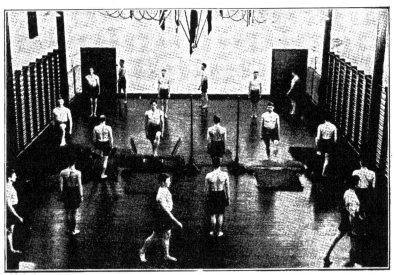

1

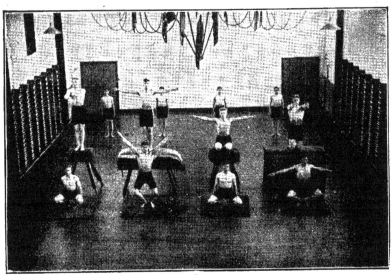

2

B. SUSPENSION EXERCISES ON APPARATUS

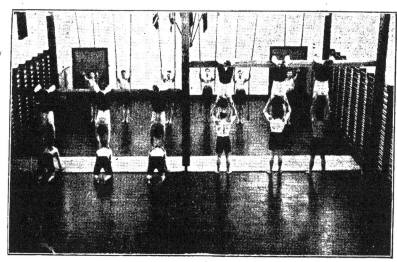

3

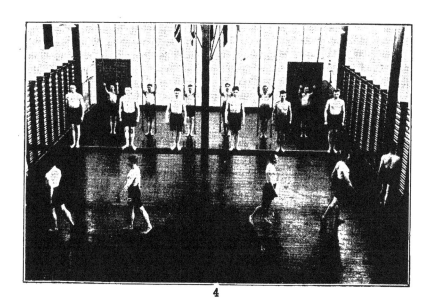

4

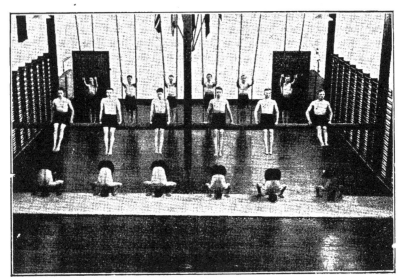

5

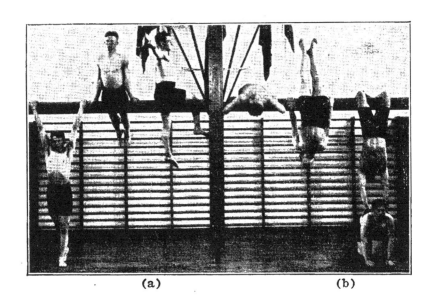

(a)   (b)

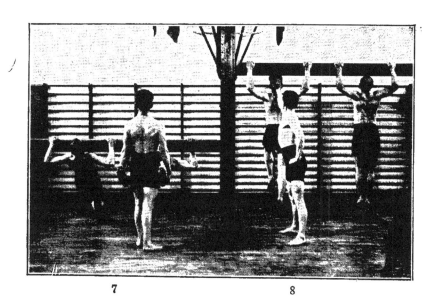

7 8

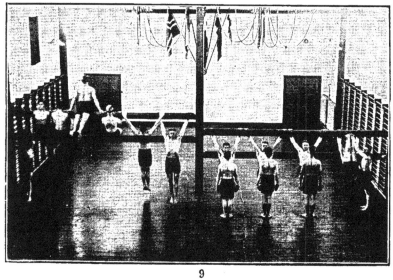

9

C. SELF TESTING ACTIVITIES ON THE MAT

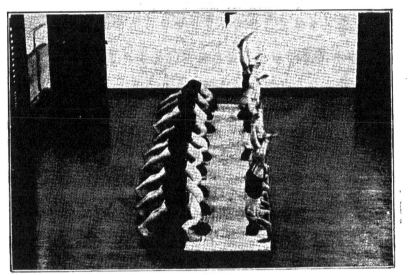

10

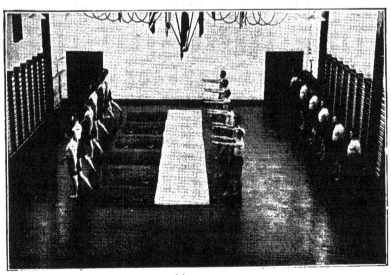

11

APPENDIX

DEFINITIONS AND EXPLANATIONS

Opposite: Facing stall bars or partner.

Side-Opposite: Side to stall bars or partner (facing same or in opposite directions).

Grasp: Hands grasping
 (1) Stall bar
 (2) Partner's hands
 (3) Any part of own body; i.e. ankles, feet, knees.

Half-Grasp: One hand grasping
 (1) Stall bar
 (2) Partner's hand
 (3) Any part of own body; i.e. ankles, feet, knees.

Support: Resting palms of hands against stall bar or partner.

(a) *Alternate:* To the left and right—alternately.
(b) *Single:* Movement taken several times to each side.

Span Bending: Active arching; back to and grasping stall bar (i.e. span-bending taken as active movement or may be helped or supported by partner after position is reached).

Chest Lifting: Active lifting of the chest (with dorsal hyper-extension), from any position.
 1. Standing
 2. Lying
 3. Kneeling
 4. Half-kneeling

Back-stretching: Rhythmical pressure downward or inward upon dorsal region—with or without help.

Trunk springing: Deep rhythmical springs of the trunk from the hip joint.

Circling: Complete circular motion—taking place in shoulder or hip joints.
  (a) In anterior-posterior plane
  (b) In diagonal-lateral plane

Flinging: A movement taking place—in shoulder or hip joints—by forceful flinging of the arms and legs to limit of range of movement.

Swinging: A movement taking place in shoulder or hip joints by an easy free swing of arms or legs from one position to another.

FORMULAE FOR NAMING STARTING POSITIONS AND MOVEMENTS

a. When an exercise is executed from the erect standing position, no starting position is named.

b. STARTING POSITIONS

Position	*Arm*	*Leg*	*Trunk*
of	Grasp or	or foot	Standing
person	support	support	Sitting
			Lying
			Hanging

Examples

Opposite —	Grasp	— Stride	Standing
Opposite —	— —	— Foot support	Long sitting
— — —	Ring—	— — — —	Back lying

c. MOVEMENTS

Speed	*Alternate* *or* *Single*	*Range*	*Movement*

Examples

Slow —   Alternate — Deep knee — Bending

The following classification and technique of indicating movements is compiled from "Gymnastic Teaching," William Skarstrom, pps. 136, 144.

1. *Combined movements:* Simultaneous movements involving two or more regions of the body. "With" connects the two parts.

2. *Alternating movements:* One movement and return to starting position followed by a second movement and return—executed alternately. "Alternating with," connects the two parts.

3. *Compound movements:* A second movement and return is interposed between two phases of the first. "And" connects the two parts.

4. *Blended compound movements:* Movements flow into each other smoothly with no definite return to a well-defined starting position. "And" (with a note of description if exercises is not clear) connects the parts.

5. *Dissimilar movements:* Given with counts.

STALL BAR EXERCISES

For the convenience of the teacher the exercises on the stall bars have been listed below. These exercises, with their necessary descriptions and signals, will be found under their own sections.

Leg Flexibility—Chapter VI

1. Grasp bow standing arm bending.
2. Grasp foot support bow lying knee stretching.
3. Bow hanging foot support knee stretching.
4. Opposite grasp half leg high standing trunk bending forward.
5. Opposite hurdle hanging trunk bending forward.[1]

Upper Back Flexibility—Chapter VI

6. Opposite grasp stride angle standing back stretching with help.
7. Stretch grasp hook lying chest lifting with help.
8. Stretch grasp knee standing back stretching with help.
9. Opposite stride angle hanging back stretching with or without help.
10. Opposite foot support long sitting back stretching with help.
11. Hanging back stretching with shoulder support or angle hanging span bending with shoulder support.
12. Hanging back stretching with foot support or angle hanging span bending with foot support.[2]
13. Opposite stretch grasp knee bow sitting back stretching with help.
14. Stretch grasp hook sitting back stretching with help.

[1] Boys' Exercise.
[2] Boys' Exercise.

LATERAL TRUNK FLEXIBILITY—CHAPTER VI

15. Side opposite foot support half standing side bending.

ARM STRENGTH—CHAPTER VII

16. Opposite support ring stride standing arm bending and stretching.
17. Opposite stride standing arm springing pushing off .from the stall bars.
18. Opposite stride angle hanging trunk lifting.
19. Stride angle hanging trunk lifting with help (wheel barrow).
20. Opposite arch hanging trunk lifting.[3]
21. Bend high hanging (feet supported) slow arm stretching.
22. Opposite grasp bow sitting trunk lifting.

NECK AND BACK STRENGTH—CHAPTER VII

23. Opposite neck hanging with support of helper.
24. Stretch grasp hook lying chest lifting.
25. Angle hanging span bending with help.
26. Angle hanging span bending.

ABDOMINAL STRENGTH—CHAPTER VII

27. Opposite foot support back angle lying trunk bending forward.
28. Hanging high knee lifting, stretching and slow sinking.

[3] Boys' Exercise.

LESSON PLANS

The principles underlying the making of lessons will be found described in detail in Chapter *III*. The following six lessons for men are translated directly, with few changes, from the original Danish edition. It is not expected that they will be taught as they appear here. Lessons must be adapted in type and rate of progression to suit class differences. The aim has been to give samples of the foregoing exercises in the book and show concretely the unique manner of building up a lesson.

These lessons may be used wholly or in part, for purposes of practice teaching, or they may suggest objectives which must be led up to by intermediate lessons.

The four lesson plans for women are not a translation. They have been planned to meet the needs of normal schools of Physical Education and colleges and could be used in any similar situation, with possibly a few changes.

They represent final objective lessons for three or four years of work. The factors which affect the progression are, time allotment and possible number of intermediate lessons. These plans must be considered in no sense a consecutive series. The tremendous gaps in progression between these four lessons presuppose carefully planned connecting lessons and efficient teaching, if the results are to be satisfactory. But the hard and fast holding of a class to the attainment of a certain final lesson results in the *teaching of exercises* and not *individuals*. The needs and abilities of a class should be the criteria in the planning.

ABBREVIATIONS USED IN LESSON PLANS

Abdominal	Abd.
Alternate	alt.
Alternating	alt'g
Arm	A.
Back	B.
Back lying	B.L.
Back stretching	B.S.
Backward	back'd
Bend	bd.
Bending	bd'g
Between	btw.
Circling	circl'g
Chest lifting	ch.l.
Clapping	clap'g
Coordination	C.
*Combined exercises	Comb.
Cross	X
Deep	dp.
Diagonally	diag'ly
Downward	down'd
Flexibility	F
Flinging	fling'g
Forward	for'd
Half	½
Hang	hg.
Hanging	hg'g
Hand	hd.
Hip joint	H.J.
Jump	jp.
Lateral	Lat.
Leg	L.
Lifting	lift'g
Lower back	L.B.

Movements	mov'ts
Neck	N.
Opposite	opp.
Placing	plac'g
Position	pos.
Quarter	¼
Raising	rais'g
Ring	rg.
Shoulder girdle	Sh.G.
Sideways	sidew.
Sideward	side'd
Sitting	sitt.
Springing	spring'g
Squat	sqt.
Standing	st.
Strength	S.
Stretching	stretch'g
Stride	strd.
Support	supp.
Swinging	swing'g
Trunk	tk.
Trunk springing	tk. spr'g
Twisting	twist'g
Upper back	U.B.
Upward	up'd
Warming up	W.
Wing	wg.
With	w.

*Combined Exercises—found in Chapter IX.

SKELETAL EXAMPLE OF A LESSON PLAN

No.	NAME OF EXERCISE	REGION	EFFECT	Ex. No.
	A.			
a 1.	....	L	W	
2.	....	A & ShG	F	
3.	....	L	C	
4.	....	A & ShG	F	
b 5.	....	L	C	
6.	....	Lat.	F	
7.	....	L & LB	F	
8.	....	A & ShG	S	
c 9.	....	L & LB	F	
10.	....	A	C	
11.	....	Lat.	F	
d 12.	....	L, LB & B	F & S	
13.	....	A & L	C	
14.	....	A	F	
15.	....	L	F	
e 16.	....	N & B	S	
17.	....	Abd.	S	
18.	....	A	S	
19.	....	Lat.	F	
20.	....	A & L	C	
	B. STALL BAR WORK			
f 21.	....	UB	F	
22.	....	L & LB	F	
23.	....	UB	F	
g 24.	....	A	S	
25.	....	Abd.	S	
	C. MARCHING, APPARATUS AND AGILITY WORK			
h 26.	March			
27.	——————			
28.	Running			
29.	Jump			
30.	——————			
i 31.	——————			
32.	——————			
33.	——————			
j 34.	Vaulting			
35.	Agility Exercises			
36.	Agility Exercises			
37.	Agility Exercises			

No.	Lesson Plan I. For Men	R	E	Ex. No.
	LESSON PLAN I. FOR MEN			
	A.			
1.	Jump in place—(lines may be opened w. these small jumps)	L	W	119
2.	Strd. st. arm fling'g btw. X & fly. . . .	A & ShG	F	30
3.	Wg. st. jump btw. strd. st. & st.	L	C	126
4.	½ wg. strd. st. single arm circl'g.	A & ShG	F	29
5.	Wg. st. easy heel rais'g & knee bd'g.	L	C	124
6.	½ wg. strd. st. tk. twist'g w. single arm fling'g	Lat.	F	53
7.	½ grasp strd. bow st. tk. spr'g	L & LB	F	11
8.	Ring hd. (supp.) strd. angle st. arm bd'g & stretch'g	A & ShG	S	76
9.	Hd. squat sitt. knee stretch'g	L & LB	F	9
10.	Double arm stretch'g up'd, sidew., for'd & down'd.	A	C	138
11.	Top strd. st. side bd'g	Lat.	F	59
12.	Neck strd. angle st. tk. spr'g & B.S. .	L,LB & B	F	22
		B	S	95
13.	Jump & hop w. alt. knee lift'g & opp. arm swing'g for'd	A & L	C	130
14.	Arm side back lying head bd'g for'd.	N	S	89
15.	Ring B.L. tk. bd'g for'd	Abd.	S	110
16.	Opp. grasp toe st. quick deep knee bd'g & stretch'g in 1 count	L	F	1
	B.			
17.	Stretch grasp hook lying ch.l. w. help	UB	F	44
18.	Grasp foot supp. bow lying knee stretch'g	L & LB	F	20
19.	Opp. grasp strd. angle st. B.S. w. help	UB	F	43
20.	Opp. supp. ring strd. st. arm bd'g & stretch'g	A	S	73
21.	Opp. strd. angle hg'g B.S. w. help. . . .	UB	F	46
22.	Opp. strd. angle hg'g tk. lift'g	A	S	81
23.	Hg'g high knee lift'g	Abd.	S	112
	C.			
24.	Free walk.			
25.	Firm walk.			
26.	Running.			
27.	High jump over low apparatus.			
28.	Preliminary jump w. double take off on low apparatus.			
29.	Running jump.			
30.	Squat vault over high apparatus.			
31.	Knee chest vault.			
32.	Standing mount on high apparatus.			
33.	Standing mount, quick dismount without pause.			
34.	Cartwheeling.			

No.	Lesson Plan II. For Men	R	E	Ex. No.
	LESSON PLAN II. FOR MEN			
	A.			
1.	Jump btw. strd. st. & st. w. hd. clap'g	A & L	W	126
2.	Arm fling'g btw. fold & arm side....	A & ShG	F	33
3.	Bd. st. 2 hops w. alt. leg fling'g sidew. w. opp. arm stretch'g sidew.......	A & L	C	127
4.	Strd. angle st. arm fling'g btw. drag & stretch.....................	A & ShG	F	34
5.	Wg. st. hop w. alt. toe touch'g sidew.	L	C	128
6.	Strd. angle st. tk. twist'g w. arm fling'g from side to side.........	Lat.	F	55
7.	Strd. angle st. arm spr'g & tk. spr'g w. hds on neck.................	A,L & LB	S, F	78
8.	'S' strd. st. side bd'g w. opp. knee bd'g............................	Lat.	F	61
9.	Heel rais'g & knee bd'g w. arm swing'g btw. reach, fold, arm side & pos...........................	A & L	C	Comb.2(f)
10.	Tk. bd'g down'd to grasp ankles....	L & LB	F	10
11.	Arm swing'g for'd & sidew. w. alt. foot plac'g sidew...............	A & L	C	120
12.	Hd. squat sitt. hop w. alt. leg stretch'g sidew..................	L & HJ	F	4
13.	Ring B.L. tk. bd'g for'd...........	Abd.	S	110
14.	B.L. alt. knee lift'g & stretch'g w. help of hds.....................	L & LB	F	17
15.	Arm side B.L. slow tk. bd'g for'd...	Abd.	S	109
16.	B.L. head bd'g for'd w. alt. knee lift'g............................	N	S	91
17.	Hd. knee st. tk. twist'g w. single arm fling'g...........................	Lat.	F	56
18.	Back clasp knee bow sitt. ch.l.......	N & B	S	98
19.	Opp. grasp strd. st. slow alt. deep knee bd'g....................	L	S	68
	B.			
20.	Stretch grasp knee st. B.S. w. help..	UB	F	45
21.	Strd. angle hg'g tk. lift'g w. help (wheelbarrow)..................	A & B	S	82
22.	Opp. stretch grasp knee bow sitt. B.S. w. help......................	UB	F	50
23.	Opp. grasp squat sitt. spring to squat sitt. on low bar..................	L & HJ	F	8
24.	Hg'g B.S. w. sh supp...............	UB	F	48
25.	Grasp bow st. arm bd'g............	L & LB	F	19
26.	Hg'g high knee lift'g & stretch'g & slow sink'g.....................	Abd.	S	112
27.	Neck supp. hg'g w. help...........	N & UB	S	93
28.	Angle hg'g span bd'g w. help.......	UB	S	104
29.	Opp. foot supp. B. angle lying (feet on 4th or 5th bar) tk. bd'g for'd to grasp stall bars.................	Abd.	S	111

No.	Lesson Plan II.—*Continued*	R	E	Ex. No.
	C.			
30.	Running.			
31.	Firm walk.			
32.	March w. turning and halting.			
33.	Toe marching.			
34.	Running jump w. turns L & R over low apparatus.			
35.	Preliminary jump over low apparatus double 'take off'.			
36.	Preliminary jump w. double 'take off' on low apparatus.			
37.	Knee chest vault over high apparatus.			
38.	Rear vault.			
39.	Oblique vault.			
40.	Head spring w. help.			
41.	Hand spring.			
42.	"Flip Flap".			
	LESSON PLAN III. FOR MEN			
	A.			
1.	Jump & hop w. alt. knee lift'g & opp. arm swing'g for'd..............	L & A	C	130
2.	⅓ wg. strd. st. single arm circl'g.....	A & ShG	F	29
3.	Wg. st. hop w. alt. toe touch'g sidew. & for'd (w. turns).........	L	C	128
4.	Arm fling'g btw. fold & arm side walking for'd & back'd.........	A & ShG	F	33
5.	Tk. bd'g down'd to grasp ankles. ..	L & LB	F	10
6.	Jump btw. squat sitt. & strd. st. w. arm rais'g sidew................	L & HJ	F	7
7.	Strd. st. tk. bd'g down'd (strik'g floor) & arm fling'g btw. drag & stretch.......................	A,L & LB	F	Comb.23
8.	Bd. st. heel rais'g & knee bd'g alt'g w. alt. knee lift'g w. arm stretch'g up'd, sidew., for'd & down'd......	L & A	C	Comb.3(e)
9.	Arm stretch'g up'd, sidew., for'd, & down'd; double, single & alt....	A	C	138
10.	Wg. st. alt. leg swing'g in circle.....	L	C	131
11.	Strd. st. tk. twist'g w. arm fling'g from side to side..............	Lat.	F	54
12.	⅓ grasp strd. bow st. tk. spr'g 4 times each side.....................	L & LB	F	11
13.	Strd. angle st. arm fling'g btw. X & fly..............................	A & ShG	F	31
14.	Hd. squat sitt. jump w. leg stretch'g sidew...........................	L & HJ	F	5

No.	Lesson Plan III.—*Continued*	R	E	Ex. No.
15.	Grasp strd. angle st. tk. spr'g.......	L & LB	F	12
16.	Neck strd. bow st. B.S. w. arm rais'g sidew.........................	N & B	S	95
17.	Ring B.L. quick tk. bd'g for'd......	Abd.	S	110
18.	Arm side B.L. ch. lift'g............	N & B	S	101
19.	Long sitt. arm fling'g btw. X & fly ..	A & ShG	F	32
20.	B.L. single & double knee lift'g & stretch'g......................	L	C	Comb.6
21.	Top ½ knee strd. st. side bd'g.......	Lat.	F	62
22.	½ knee st. tk. bd'g for'd w. straightening of for'd knee..............	L & LB	F	15
23.	4 hops w. alt. leg swing'g for'd & back'd w. arm swing'g for'd & sidew............................	L & A	C	132
24.	Side opp. grasp strd. twist st. arm swing'g outw. & up'd...........	A & ShG	F	37
25.	½ grasp strd. bow st. tk. spr'g changing w. twist..................	L & LB	F	11
26.	Opp. grasp strd. st. slow alt. deep knee bd'g.....................	L	S	68
	B.			
27.	Opp. foot supp. long sitt. B.S. w. help............................	UB	F	47
28.	Opp. foot supp. long sitt. tk. spr'g w. help......................	L & LB	F	24
29.	Opp. foot supp. long sitt. arm circl'g w. help......................	A & ShG	F	38
30.	Opp. foot supp. strd. long sitt. lift'g of hips w. supp. of helper........	N & B	S	94
31.	Hg'g B.S. w. shoulder supp........	UB	F	48
32.	Bow hg'g foot supp. knee stretch'g ..	L & LB	F	21
33.	Hg'g single & double knee lift'g & stretch'g & slow sink'g..........	Abd.	S	112
34.	Opp. arch hg'g tk. lift'g..........	A	S	83
35.	Opp. grasp squat sitt. spring to squat sitt. pos. on low bar...........	L & HJ	F	8
36.	Bd. high hg'g slow arm stretch'g....	A	S	84
37.	Angle hg'g span bd'g w. help.......	B	S	104
38.	Grasp bow st. arm bd'g............	L & LB	F	19
39.	Hd. st. w. supp..................	A	S	80
	C.			
40.	Marching and turning.			
41.	Firm walk.			
42.	Marching sideways.			
43.	Running jump over low apparatus w. arm rais'g sidew.			
44.	Preliminary jump w. single foot take off from low apparatus.			
45.	Squat vault over high apparatus.			
46.	Rear vault crosswise.			

No.	LESSON PLAN III.—*Continued*	R	E	Ex. No.
47.	Oblique vault w. turn.			
48.	Rear vault over high apparatus (lengthwise).			
49.	Straddle vault (apparatus lengthwise).			
50.	Head spring.			
51.	Hand spring.			
52.	Backward rolls.			

LESSON PLAN IV. FOR MEN

A.

No.		R	E	Ex. No.
1.	Jump btw. strd. st. & st. w. one jump in place w. hd. clap'g overhead...	L & A	W	Comb.1(b)
2.	Heel rais'g & knee bd'g w. arm fling'g btw. X & fly.............	L,A,ShG	F	Comb.2(g)
3.	Wg. st. 4 hops w. alt. toe touch'g sidew. & knee lift'g & toe touch'g for'd & knee lift'g..............	L	C	133
4.	Strd. angle st. arm fling'g btw. drag & stretch.....................	A & ShG	F	34
5.	½ wg. strd. st. tk. twist'g w. single arm fling'g.....................	Lat.	F	53
6.	½ grasp strd. bow st. tk. spr'g......	L & LB	F	11
7.	Strd. angle st. tk. twist'g w. arm fling'g from side to side..........	Lat.	F	55
8.	Bd. st. hop w. alt. toe touch'g sidew. & for'd w. arm stretch'g sidew. & for'd...........................	L & A	C	128
9.	'S' strd. st. side bd'g of tk. w. opp. knee bd'g.....................	Lat.	F	61
10.	Neck strd. angle st. tk. spr'g.......	L & LB	F	22
11.	Hd. squat sitt. knee stretch'g w. tk. spr'g........................	L & LB	F	23
12.	Bow st. trunk rais'g ch.l. w. low hd. turning......................	N & B	S	99
13.	Alt. leg swing'g for'd & back'd w. hd. clap'g.....................	L & A	C	135
14.	Hd. squat sitt. hop w. alt. leg stretch'g sidew..................	L & HJ	F	4
15.	Ring B.L. quick tk. bd'g for'd......	Abd.	S	110
16.	Arm side B.L. head bd'g for'd alt'g w. ch. lift'g....................	N & UB	S	101
17.	B.L. alt. knee lift'g & stretch'g w. arm stretch'g up'd, sidew., for'd & down'w......................	L & A	C	Comb.6
18.	Hurdle sitt. tk. bd'g for'd...........	L & LB	F	16
19.	Hd. knee st. tk. twist'g w. single arm fling'g.....................	Lat.	F	56
20.	Front lying ch.l. w. arm rais'g sidew.	N & B	S	100

No.	Lesson Plan IV.—*Continued*	R	E	Ex. No.
21.	Strd. front lying hip rais'g w. arm stretch'g.....................	Abd.	S	113
22.	Wg. st. quick heel rais'g & deep knee bd'g...........................	L & HJ	F	3
23.	Strd. st. quick tk. bd'g down'd (strik'g floor) & arm fling'g btw. drag & stretch.................	L,LB & A	F	Comb.23
24.	Easy heel rais'g & knee bd'g w. arm swing'g for'd & sidew. & circl'g...	L & A	C	Comb.2(c)
25.	Hd. st. w. supp.....................	A	S	80
26.	Opp. knee sitt. back'd bd'g of tk. w. supp. of helper................	Abd.	S	116
27.	Opp. foot supp. ring B.L. (legs locked) quick tk. bd'g for'd.....	Abd.	S	108
28.	Heel rais'g & knee bd'g alt'g w. alt. knee lift'g w. arm stretch'g up'd, sidew., for'd & down'd; double, single & alt.....................	L & A	C	Comb.3(e)
	B.			
29.	Opp. strd. angle hg'g B.S. w. help...	UB	F	46
30.	Opp. strd. angle hg'g tk. lift'g......	A & B	S	81
31.	Opp. grasp strd. st. B.S. w. help....	UB	F	43
32.	Opp. bow hg'g tk. lift'g............	A & B	S	86
33.	Stretch grasp hook bow sitt. B.S. w. help............................	UB	F	51
34.	Opp. foot supp. long sitt. tk. spr'g w. help............................	L & LB	F	24
35.	Opp. foot supp. B. angle lying tk. bd'g for'd to grasp stall bar......	Abd.	S	111
36.	Hg'g B.S. w. foot supp.............	UB	F	49
37.	Grasp bow st. arm bd'g............	L & LB	F	19
38.	Opp. stretch grasp knee bow sitt. B.S. w. help....................	UB	F	50
39.	Hg'g high knee lift'g & stretch'g & slow sink'g....................	Abd.	S	112
40.	Walking on hds.			
	C.			
41.	Free walk			
42.	Running			
43.	Marching w. turning			
44.	" Kick " walk			
45.	Knee chest vault w. turns			
46.	High jump over high apparatus			
47.	" Thief " vault			
48.	Rear vault lengthwise			
49.	Straddle vault lengthwise			
50.	Hd. spring over low apparatus			
51.	Head spring w. jump & turn & back'd roll w. jump & turn			
52.	"Flip Flap"			
53.	Hd. spring followed by head spring			
54.	"Flying somersault"			

No.	LESSON PLAN V. FOR MEN	R	E	Ex. No.
	LESSON PLAN V. FOR MEN			
	A.			
1.	4 hops w. alt. leg swing'g for'd & back'd w. arm swing'g for'd & sidew....................	L & A	C	132
2.	Arm circl'g in opp. directions (1 for'd, 1 back'd)................	A	F	35
3.	Jump btw. strd. st. & st. w. 2 jumps in place w. arm rais'g sidew., bd'g & stretch'g down'd...............	L & A	C	126
4.	Walk'g for'd & back'd w. arm fling'g btw. fold & side arm..........	A	F	33
5.	Jump from squat sitt. to strd. st. & one jump in place w. hd. clap'g over head	L & A	C	134
6.	Tk. bd'g down'd to grasp ankles w. arm bd'g & tk. rais'g & arm stretch'g over head, sidew. down'd	L & LB	F	10
7.	Heel rais'g & knee bd'g w. arm swing'g for'd & sidew. & circl'g. ..	L & A	C	Comb.3(b)
8.	'S' strd. st. side bd'g w. opp. knee bd'g (4 times each side)..........	S	F	61
9.	Neck strd. angle st. tk. spr'g.......	L & LB	F	22
10.	Ring hd. strd. angle st. arm bd'g & stretch'g.....................	A & ShG	S	76
11.	Hd. knee st. tk. twist'g w. single arm fling'g.........................	S	F	56
12.	Top ¼ squat strd. sitt. side bd'	S	F	63
13.	Hd. squat sitt. hop w. alt. leggstr'g sidew........................	L	F	4
14.	Arm side B.L. slow tk. bd'g for'd:...	Abd.	S	109
15.	Grasp hook sitt. head circl'g........	N	F	42
16.	Neck long bow sitt. ch.l. w. low hd. turning......................	N & B	S	96
17.	B.L. alt. knee stretch'g w. help of hds............................	L	F	17
18.	Ring B.L. quick tk. bd'g for'd......	Abd.	S	110
19.	B. clasp knee bow sitt. ch.l. w. arm rais'g sidew...................	N & B	S	98
20.	Opp. knee st. tk. bd'g back'd w. supp. of helper.................	Abd.	S	116
21.	Hd. squat sitt. knee stretch'g.......	L & LB	F	9
22.	Heel rais'g & knee bd'g alt'g w. knee lift'g.........................	L & A	C	123 & 124
23.	Top strd. st. single knee bd'g & stretch'g pushing off w. side bd'g..	L & S	S & F	69
24.	Hd. st. arm bd'g w. help..........	A & ShG	S	80
25.	Opp. grasp squat sitt. hop w. alt. leg stretch'g for'd...............	L	F	6
26.	Opp. foot supp. long sitt. B.S. w. help............................	UB	F	47

No.	Lesson Plan V.—*Continued*	R	E	
27.	Opp. foot supp. long sitt. tk. spring'g w. help......................	L & LB	F	24
28.	Opp. foot supp. long sitt. arm circl'g w. help......................	S	F	38
29.	Neck B. angle lying leg swing'g from side to side w. supp. of helper.	Lat.	S	118
30.	Opp. foot supp. strd. long sitt. lift'g of hips w. supp. of helper........	N & B	S	94
	B.			
31.	Stretch grasp knee st. B.S. w. help..	UB	F	45
32.	Opp. stretch grasp knee bow sitt. B.S. w. help...................	UB	F	50
33.	Hg'g single & double knee lift'g & stretch'g & slow sink'g..........	Abd.	S	112
34.	Grasp bow st. arm bd'g...........	L & LB	F	19
35.	'S' side opp. foot supp. ½ st. side bd'...........................	S	F	64
36.	Angleghg'g span bd'g.............	N & B	S	105
37.	Opp. long sitt. tk. bd'g for'd to grasp feet........................	L	F	13
	C.			
38.	Hg'g B.S. over double boom.			
39.	Over grasp hg'g arm bd'g			
40.	Grasp st. for'd swing on ropes to side sitt. on boom.			
41.	Grasp st. for'd swing on ropes to knee hg'g on boom.			
42.	Grasp st. for'd swing on ropes to st. on boom.			
43.	Free balance walk on boom at hip level			
44.	Alt. free walk and light marching			
45.	Running w. changing steps.			
46.	March w. leg swing.			
47.	St. mount & deep jump dismount w. out a pause on high apparatus (crosswise.)			
48.	Squat vault over high apparatus (crosswise.)			
49.	Straddle vault over high apparatus (lengthwise.)			
50.	B. vault w. turns over high apparatus (lengthwise.)			
52.	Hd. spring over high apparatus (crosswise.)			
53.	Head spring turn about jump back'd roll turning about jump.			
54.	Hd. spring followed by fly somersault.			
55.	Flip flap			
56.	Flying somersault.			

No.	Lesson Plan VI. For Men	R	E	Ex. No.
	LESSON PLAN VI. FOR MEN			
	A.			
1.	Jump in place w. arm stretch'g up'd, sidew. for'd & down'd, double, single & alternate...............	L & A	C	119 & 138
2.	Jump & hop w. alt. knee lift'g & opp. arm swing'g for'd..............	L & A	C	130
3.	Wg. st. 2 hops w. alt. leg fling'g sidew......................	L	C	127
4.	Bd. st. hop w. alt. toe touch'g sidew. & for'd w. arm stretch'g sidew. & for'd........................	L & A	C	128
5.	Walking for'd & back'd w. arm fling'g btw. fold & arm side......	A	F	33
6.	Tk. bd'g down'd to grasp ankles....	L & LB	F	10
7.	Jump from squat sitt. to strd. st. w. 3 jumps in place w. arm mov'ts...	L & A	S & F	Comb.14
8.	Strd. st. tk. bd'g down'd (strike floor) & arm fling'g btw. drag & stretch......................	A	F	Comb.23
9.	Jump btw. strd. st. & st. w. hd. clap'g 5 times & 5 jumps in place.	L & A	C	126
10.	Heel rais'g & knee bd'g w. arm swing'g for'd & sidew. (hold'g one arm 1 count every 4th count)....	L & A	C	Comb.2(f)
11.	Strd. st. arm circl'g in opp. direction.	A	F	35
12.	Heel rais'g & knee bd'g alt'g w. knee lift'g w. arm stretch'g up'd, sidew. for'd & down'd; double, single & alternate......................	L & A	C	Comb.3(e)
13.	Jump btw. strd. st. & st. w. one jump in place w. arm placing—sidew. bd'g up'd—placing sidew., bd'g, for'd—sidew., bd'g down'd.......	L & A	C	Comb.1(k)
14.	Heel rais'g & knee bd'g alt'g w. alternate knee lift'g w. arm fling'g btw. X & fly.....................	A	F	Comb.2(g)
15.	Heel rais'g & knee bd'g & alt. knee lift'g w. arm swing'g btw. reach, fold, arm side, pos. & in reverse order......................	L & A	C	Comb.2(j)
16.	½ wg. strd. st. tk. twist'g w. single arm fling'g.....................	UB	F	53
17.	½ grasp strd. bow st. tk. spr'g......	L & LB	F	11
18.	Strd. angle st. tk. twist'g w. arm fling'g........................	S	F	55
19.	Neck strd. angle st. tk. spr'g.......	L & LB	F	22
20.	S strd. st. side bd'g w. opp. knee bd'g	S	F	61
21.	Heel rais'g & knee bd'g w. arm swing'g for'd & sidew. & circl'g...	L & A	C	Comb.2(c)
22.	Hd. squat sitt. knee stretch'g w. tk. spr'g........................	L & LB	F	23

No.	LESSON PLAN VI.—*Continued*	R	E	Ex. No.
23.	Alt. leg swing'g for'd & back'd w. hd. clap'g...............	L & A	C	135
24.	Knee st. arm spring'g & arm fling'g .	A	S & F	77
25.	Front lying leg & chest lift'g w. arm rais'g sidew...................	N & UB	S	100
26.	Strd. front lying hip raising.......	Abd.	S	113
27.	Bd. st. 4 hops w. alt. toe touch'g sidew. & knee lift'g & toe touch'g for'd & knee lift'g.............	L & A	C	133
28.	Side opp. grasp strd. twist st. arm fling'g out'd ' up'd.............	A	F	37
29.	½ grasp strd. bow st. tk. spring'g changing w. twist.............	L & LB	F	11
30.	Knee st. tk. bd'g back'd w. supp. of helper.......................	Abd. & B	S & F	116
31.	Opp. ½ grasp strd. st. slow alt. deep knee bd'g w. turns w. opp. arm rais'g diag'ly up'd.............	L	S	71
	B.			
32.	Stretch grasp B.L. ch.l. w. help......	UB	F	44
33.	Grasp foot supp. bow lying knee stretch'g....................	L & LB	F	20
34.	Hang'g B.S. w. foot supp.........	UB	F	49
35.	Grasp bow st. arm bd'g.........	L & LB	F	19
36.	Opp. grasp squat sitt.—spring to squat sitt. on low bar..........	L	F	8
37.	Bd. high hang'g slow arm stretch'g w. knee lift'g.................	A & B	S	84
38.	Stretch grasp long sitt. span bd'g alt'g w. tk. bd'g for'd to grasp feet......................	N & B	S	105
39.	Hang'g leg swing'g to foot supp. bow hang'g knee stretch'g...........	Abd.	S	112
40.	Hd. st., span bd'g...............	N & B	S	106
	C.			
41.	Boom: under grasp back'd circle to sitt. back rest w. back circle to inverted hg'g, knee hanging, hd. st. dismount.			
42.	Over grasp hg'g arm bd'g.			
43.	Balance walk on boom over head high.			
44.	For'd swing to st. on boom.			
45.	For'd swing to sitt. on boom dismount followed by head spring.			
46.	For'd swing to knee hg'g dismount hd. supp. from another man's back.			
47.	Free walk.			
48.	Marching sidew. w. turn to toe marching back'd & for'd.			
49.	Running w. turning about to run back'd.			

No.	LESSON PLAN VI.—*Continued*	R	E	Ex. No.
50.	Light march.			
51.	Kick march & turn.			
52.	March w. leg swing'g.			
53.	High jump over high apparatus.			
54.	High hand spring.			
55.	Rear straddle vault.			
56.	Hand spring over low apparatus & hand st. walk off mat.			
57.	Head spring two or three quickly after each other.			
58.	Hand spring & head spring.			
59.	Hand spring & flying somersault.			
60.	Flying somersault.			

No.	Lesson Plan I. For Women	R	E	Ex. No.
	LESSON PLAN I. FOR WOMEN			
	A.			
1.	Jp. in place w. arm stretch'g upw'd sidew. for'd & down'd..........	L & A	C & W	119 & 138
2.	½ wg. strd. st. single arm circl'g.....	A & ShG	F	29
3.	Strd. st. arm fling'g btw. X & fly...	A & ShG	F	30
4.	Jp. btw. sqt. sitt. & strd. st........	L & HJ	F	7
5.	Hd. sqt. sitt. knee stretch'g.......	L & LB	F	9
6.	Alt. leg swing'g for'd & back'd w. hd. clap'g......................	L & A	C	135
7.	Alt. foot plac'g sidew. w. arm swing'g for'd and sidew...............	L & A	C	120 & 140
8.	'S' strd. ½ toe st. side bd'g........	Lat.	F	60
9.	Hd. half sqt. strd. sitt. (pushing off w. hds.) alt. knee str'g & bd'g....	L	S	70
10.	Strd. st. trunk twist'g w. arm fling'g from side to side...............	Lat.	F	54
11.	Rg. back lying quick trunk bd'g for'd	Abd.	S	110
12.	Long sitt. arm fling'g btw. X & fly..	A & ShG	F	32
13.	Grasp hook bow sitt. chest lift'g....	N & B	S	97
14.	Grasp hook sitt. head turning, bd'g, & circl'g......................	N	F	39
15.	Back lying alt. knee bd'g & stretch'g w. arm bd'g & stretch'g upw'd & down'd......................	L & A	C	Comb. 6
16.	Grasp ½ hook lying head bd'g for'd alt'g w. ch. l.	N & B	S	90 & 102
17.	B.L. alt. knee lift'g & stretch'g w. help of hands..................	L	F	17
18.	Hd. knee st. trunk twist'g w. single arm fling'g..................	Lat.	F	56
19.	Rg. hd. knee st. arm bd'g & stretch'g.	A	S	75
20.	Knee st. arm swing'g for'd & sidew..	A	C	140
21.	Opp. grasp st. (w. partner) slow heel rais'g & dp. knee bd'g..........	L	S	66
	B.			
22.	Opp. strd. angle st. B.S. w. help....	UB	F	46
23.	Grasp bow st. arm bd'g....	L & UB	F	19
24.	Opp. foot supp. back angle lying tr'k bd'g for'd to grasp stall bar.	Abd.	S	111
25.	Opp. strd. st. arm spring'g from bar.	A	S	74
	LESSON PLAN II. FOR WOMEN			
	A.			
1.	Bd. st. hop w. alt. toe touch'g sidew. and for'd w. arm str'g sidew. and for'd......................	L & A	C.W.	128
2.	Wg. st. easy heel rais'g & knee bd'g w. arm swing'g for'd and sidew. ..	L & A	C	124 & 140

No.	Lesson Plan II.—*Continued*	R	E	Ex. No.
3.	Strd. st. arm fling'g btw. X & fly w. heel rais'g....................	A	F	30
4.	Neck strd. bow st. trunk spr'g & back stretch'g................	L & LB	F	22
5.	Hd. squat sitt. knee stretch'g w. spring'g.....................	L & LB	F	9
6.	Jump from squat sitt. to strd. st. & st. w. hd. clap'g...............	L & A	C	134
7.	Alt. toe touch'g sidew. w. arm swing'g for'd & sidew. & side bd'g (4 times w. arms in 'S').........	Lat.	F	60
8.	Alt. knee lift'g & stretch'g w. help of hds......................	L	F	18
9.	½ wg. strd. st. trunk twist'g w. single arm fling'g....................	Lat.	F	53
10.	½ grasp strd. bow st. trunk spr'g....	L & LB	F	11
11.	Strd. angle st. w. arm fling'g btw. drag & stretch.................	A	F	34
12.	Jp. in place w. any arm movement desired......................	L	C	119
13.	Bd. st. single knee bd'g & stretch'g pushing off w. arm stretch'g sidew..	L	S	69
14.	Long sitt. tk. bd'g for'd to grasp ankles & arm bd'g..............	L & LB	F	13
15.	Arm side B.L. head & alt. knee lift'g.	N & B	S	89 & 123
16.	Arm side hook lying ch.l...........	B	S	101
17.	B.L. alt. knee str'g w. help of hds...	L	F	17
18.	Hook sitt. (hds. free on floor beside knees) alternate & double arm fling'g for'd & up'd.............	A	F	36
19.	Grasp hook bow sitt. (hds. on knees) ch.l. w. arm rais'g sidew.........	UB	S	97
20.	Hd. knee st. trunk twist'g w. single arm fling'g....................	Lat.	F	56
21.	Ring hd. knee st. arm bd'g alt'g w. knee stretch'g.................	A	S	75
22.	Back clasp knee bow sitt. ch.l...... ..	N & B	S	98
23.	Knee st. arm swing'g for'd & sidew. w. alt. leg stretch'g sidew........	L & A	C	140
24.	4 hops w. alt. leg swing'g for'd & back'd w. arm swing'g for'd & sidew......................	L & A	C	132 & 140
25.	Opp. grasp strd. st. slow alt. deep knee bd'g.....................	L	S	68
26.	Opp. grasp st. hop w. alt. toe touch'g sidew. & quick deep knee bd'g.....	L & A	C	Comb.16
27.	Opp. ring B.L. (legs locked) tk. bd'g for'd......................	Abd.	S	108
28.	Opp. grasp hook sitt. (pull to st.)...	......	......	......
	B.			
29.	Opp. strd. angle hg'g B.S. w. help...	UB	F	46
30.	Opp. strd. angle hg'g tr. lift'g......	A	S	81

No.	LESSON PLAN II.—*Continued*	R	E	Ex. No.
31.	Opp. foot supp. long sitt. B.S. w. help	UB	F	47
32.	Opp. foot supp. long sitt. tk. spring'g w. help......................	L & LB	F	24
33.	Opp. foot supp. long sitt. arms circl'g w. help..................	A & ShG	F	38
34.	Stretch grasp st. alt. & double high knee lift'g, stretch'g & slow sink'g.	Abd.	S	114
35.	Opp. grasp squat sitt. spring to a squat sitt. pos. on low bar.......	L	F	8
	LESSON PLAN III. FOR WOMEN			
	A.			
1.	Alt. heel rais'g w. opp. arm swing'g for'd & back'd..................	L & A	C & W	
2.	Jump & hop w. alt. knee lift'g & opp. arm swing'g for'd..............	L & A	C	130
3.	Bd. st. 2 hops w. alt. leg fling'g sidew. w. arm stretch'g up'd & sidew.........................	L & A	C	Comb.5(c)
4.	Heel rais'g & knee bd'g w. arm fling'g btw. X & fly, several times, on signal change w. jump to —......	L & A	F	Comb.2(g)
5.	Strd. st. arm fling'g btw. X & fly...	A	F	30
6.	Grasp bow st. arm bd'g & tk. rais'g & ch.l..........................	B	S	99
7.	Arm swing'g for'd & sidew.........	A	C	140
8.	Hd. squat sitt. knee stretch'g w. tk. spr'g & arm fling'g btw. X & fly..	L,LB,Sh,A	F	Comb.24
9.	Strd. angle st. tk. twist'g w. arm fling'g from side to side.........	Lat.	F	54
10.	½ grasp strd. bow st. tk. spr'g (change w. twist).....................	L & LB	F	11
11.	'S' strd. st. side bd'g w. single opp. knee bd'g....................	Lat.	F	61
12.	Jump btw. strd. st. & st. & turning w. one jump in place w. arm plac'g sidew. bd'g stretch'g up'd, plac'g sidew. bd'g & stretch'g down'd...	L & A	C	Comb.1(k)
13.	Hd. squat sitt. hop w. alt. leg stretch'g sidew. (5cts) & jump w. double leg stretch'g back'd (2cts)..	L,LB,Abd.	F & S	Comb.30
14.	Ring B.L. quick tk. bd'g for'd......	Abd.	S	110
15.	Grasp ½ hook lying head bd'g for'd alt'g w. ch.l...................	N & B	S	90
16.	B.L. alt. & double knee lift'g & stretch'g w. arm bd'g & stretch'g —up'd, sidew., for'd & down'd...	L & A	C	Comb.6
17.	Arm side B.L. slow tk. bd'g for'd...	Abd.	S	109
18.	Grasp long bow sitt. leg lift'g w. help of hds....................	L & LB	F	14

No.	Lesson Plan III.—*Continued*	R	E	Ex. No.
19.	Hurdle sitt. tk. bd'g for'd..........	L & LB	F	16
20.	Long sitt. arm fling'g btw. X & fly & tk. spring'g (4 times each).....	A.L & LB	F	32
21.	Neck hook bow sitt. ch.l...........	N & B	S	97
22.	Ring hd. knee st. (one leg rais'd high) arm bd'g................	A	S	75
23.	½ knee st. tk. bd'g for'd w. straightening of for'd knee................	L & LB	F	15
24.	Knee st. arm swing'g for'd & sidew. w. alt. leg stretch'g sidew. & side bd'g (w. arms in S)............	Lat.	F	62
25.	Knee st. arm swing'g for'd & sidew..	A	C	140
26.	Reach squat sitt. arm parting & slow knee stretch'g w. arm lower'g to side........................	L	S	
27.	Jump & alt. heel touch'g for'd & toe touch'g in place w. arm mov'ts...	L & A	C	Comb.10
28.	Opp. ½ grasp strd. st. slow alt. deep knee bd'g w. alt. arm rais'g diag'ly sidew. up'd.............	L	S	71
29.	Neck back angle lying leg swing'g from side to side w. supp. of helper......................	Lat.	S	118
30.	Opp. foot supp. strd. long sitt. lift'g of hips w. supp. of helper....	N & B	S	94
	B.			
31.	Stretch grasp hook lying ch.l. w. help & leg swing'g to bar over head & knee stretch'g & tk. bd'g for'd to grasp ankles..................	UB & L	F	44 & 20
32.	Bd. high hg'g slow arm stretch'g....	A	S	84
33.	Opp. stretch grasp knee bow sitt. B.S. w. help....................	UB	F	50
34.	Opp. grasp bow sitt. tk. lift'g.......	A & B	S	85
35.	Angle hg'g span bd'g w. help.......	B	S	104
	LESSON PLAN IV. FOR WOMEN			
	A.			
1.	Jp. in place w. arm stretch'g up'd sidew. for'd & down'd, double single and alternate.............	L & A	C	119 & 138
2.	Hop w. alt. toe touch'g sidew. turn'g & for'd w. quick deep knee bend'g w. arm stretch'g sidew. & for'd...	L & A	C	Comb.16
3.	½ wg. st. alt. foot placing sidew. w. single arm swing'g for'd & back'd (2 cts.) & single arm circl'g (5 times) 6 counts each side........	A	F	29

No.	Lesson Plan IV.—*Continued*	R	E	Ex. No.
4.	Wg. st. heel rais'g & knee bd'g & alt. knee lift'g w. arm swing'g btw. reach, fold, arm side, position, and in reverse order........	L & A	C	Comb-3 (j.) & ex. 23)
5.	Top st. single foot plac'g sidew. & knee bend'g & stretch'g pushing off w. side bend'g..............	L & Lat.	S & F	69
6.	2 hops w. alt. leg fling'g sidew. w. arm stretch'g up'd, for'd, sidew. & down'd.....................	L & A	C	Comb.5
7.	Walking for'd & back'd (6 cts.) w. arm fling'g btw. fold & arm side & tk. spring'g (4 times).........	A	F	33
8.	Head bd'g for'd w. alt. knee lift'g (hds. grasp'g knees) & tk. bd'g down'd to grasp ankles w. arm bd'g fol. by tk. rais'g w. ch.l. w. arm stretch'g slowly over head, sidew. down'd	L & LB	Comb.	27
9.	Jump from squat sitt. to stride st. & st. with arm movements.......	L & A	Comb.	14
10.	Heel rais'g & knee bd'g w. arm swing'g & circl'g & alt. foot placing sidew. & side bend'g........	A & L Lat.	Comb. Series	2
11.	½ wg. stride st. tk. twist'g w. arm fling'g (changing every 4 times) ...	Lat.	F	53
12.	Grasp stride bow st. tk. stretch'g for'd w. arm rais'g sidew.........	B	S	95
13.	4 hops w. alt. toe touch'g sidew. & knee lift'g & toe touch'g for'd & knee l. & a quick deep knee bend'g fol. by a ½ turn L or R w. arm movements...................	L & A	Comb.	9
14.	Grasp long bow sitt. ch.l. w. slow arm stretch'g up'd, sidew. & down'd..	N & B	S	96
15.	Grasp long bow sitt. arm bd'g & slow back'd bd'g of tk. w. arm placing sidew. alt'g w. (hd. side foot lying) hip rais'g w. single arm rais'g sidew. up'd..............	Lat.	S	117
16.	Arm side B.L. head & alt. knee lift'g alt'g w. chest, arm & leg left'g....	B	Comb.	22
17.	Arm side B.L. slow tk. bd'g for'd to hook sitt. (hds. grasp ankles) single & double knee stretch'g....	L	Comb.	20
18.	Arm side B.L. slow tk. bd'g for'd to angle sitt. arm rais'g sidew. (see illustration 115)...............	Abd.	S	115
19.	Long sitt. arm fling'g btw. fold & arm side...........................	A	F	32
20.	Hand knee st. tk. twist'g w. alt. arm fling'g........................	Lat.	F	56

No.	LESSON PLAN IV.—*Continued*	R	E	Ex. No.
21.	Stride front lying hip rais'g	Abd.	S	113
22.	Front lying chest, arm & leg lift'g . . .	B	S	100
23.	Knee st. arm spring'g, arm fling'g btw. X & fly.	A	S	77
24.	Knee st. arm swing'g for'd & sidew. (stand'g) heel rais'g & knee bd'g w. arm swing'g for'd sidew. (holding one arm one ct. every 4th ct.) . .	A	Comb.	2 (f)
25.	Opp. grasp foot supp. hook sitt. alt. & double leg stretch'g & tk. pulling for'd.	B	S	87
26.	Opp. foot supp. long sitt. tk. rais'g w. supp. of helper.	N & B	S	94
27.	Side opp. grasp strd. twist. st. arm swing'g sidew. up'd.	A.ShG	F	37
28.	Side opp. strd. angle st. arm fling'g btw. drag & stretch.	A.ShG	F	34
29.	Repeat No. 28 after changing direction w. 3 little jumps (one in strd. & two in place).	A.ShG	F	37
30.	Side opp. ¼ grasp strd. bow st. tk. spring'g, chang'g w. twist	L & LB	F	11
	B.			
31.	Opp. stride angle hg'g B.S. w.out help.	UB	F	43
32.	Opp. strd. angle hg'g tk. lift'g	A & B	S	81
33.	Angle hg'g leg swing'g over head w. help (to bow hg'g knee stretch'g) . .	L & HJ	F	21
34.	Side opp. foot supp. half st. S.B.	Lat.	F	64
35.	Span bend'g w.out help.	B	S	105

TESTS OF IMPROVEMENT IN FUNDAMENTAL GYMNASTICS

The following tests have been used for three years at the Central School of Hygiene and Physical Education. They consist of certain specific exercises measuring arm and leg flexibility; arm, leg, and abdominal strength; and two agility tests. One of the agility tests involves a jump over a piece of apparatus and the other includes an element of speed, with a quick change of body position.

The purpose of these tests is twofold: (1) To graphically interest the student in his own improvement in relation to the other members of his class and: (2) To provide an excellent guide for the teacher in determining the homogeneity of her group and the rate of improvement in flexibility, strength and agility.

In so far as possible, the attempt has been made to eliminate the element of judgment. This has not been entirely successful but by carefully controlling the procedure, and scoring by zones, much of this difficulty is overcome.

Scores and a rating table are given here only to show the possibility of such a procedure, but it is advocated that each teacher make some such tables from her own statistics and rate her pupils by them.

It seems impractical, at present, to get a standard rating by compiling results from different schools, because of the difficulty in deciding on a uniform method of giving the tests that will eliminate the possibility of differences in technique and judgment. With a little practice, a teacher can give these tests to her own classes so quickly and with such great uniformity that the gain indicated throughout the year will be a very accurate index of the general improvement. A back strength test is now being used but the results have not yet been determined.

In submitting these tests it is earnestly hoped there will be no misunderstanding regarding them. They must not be considered, in any sense, as scientific motor ability tests. They merely, in a general way, indicate improvement during a course in Fundamental Gymnastics. They are still being used experimentally and do not represent an exhaustive or finished study of the material. Because of this they are offered here with a great feeling of hesitancy and only because of the evident interest in and demand for them from all sections of the country.

A chart, recording scores of individual and class improvement, is a possible means for stimulating interest. Such a chart is included here merely as a sample of the procedure, also, it will be noted, that no score falls below a score of 6. In a highly selected normal school group, for whom these tests were planned, no score fell below this mark. However, this undoubtedly will not be the case in other groups.

DESCRIPTION AND METHOD OF GIVING TESTS

a. To Measure Flexibility

1. *Arm and shoulder girdle*

'Arm flinging between X and fly.' Chapter VI. Ex. 30.

Procedure:

Have student heel one of the lines in front of wall or stall bars. Let him try to touch same in performing arm flinging—wrists straight—fingers clenched—without leaning backward. Instructor stands at side and watches posture of student in arm flinging—chest out—head back—action free.

Instruction:

Explain test simply and do not urge the pupil on. Warn him against knocking his fingers when standing close to the wall.

2. *Leg*

(Stall bars)

'Grasp bow standing arm bending.' Chapter VI. Ex. 19.

Procedure:

Have student stand with back to stall bars (gastrocnemius just touching), and grasp lowest bar possible without bending knees —trying to approximate trunk to thighs. Instructor stands at side and watches student.

Instruction:

Explain test carefully. Do not urge student on—(liability of strain to lower back). Be sure knees are straight and legs are touching bar. (Have another student stand in front of person taking test, in case he loses his balance.)

b. TO MEASURE STRENGTH

1. *Arms*

'Bend high hanging slow arm stretching against time.' Chapter VII. Ex. 84.

Procedure:

Have student climb bars and hang facing outward. Elbow joints should form right angles. Grasp bar so that head is over smooth intersection between the stall bars, or insert a board over the ribs of the stall bars.

Instruction:

Explain simply—be sure elbows and shoulder joints are correct, and do not stimulate. See that pupil's feet are removed from support of bar before starting stop-watch.

2. *Leg*

'Opposite grasp wide stride standing alternate slow deep knee bending.' Chapter VII. Ex. 68.

Procedure:

Have student choose a partner of about the same height (or instructor works with pupil) and they stand close together.

Instruction:

Explain that the movement is slow and executed with complete knee bending, making the change from one side to the other without jerks, and with back straight and knees well turned out.

3. *Abdomen*

(Stall bars)—'Stretch grasp standing single and double high knee lifting and stretching and slow sinking.' Chapter VII. Ex. 114.

Procedure:

Arrange stool or bench in such a way that student may grasp highest bar and still have his feet or toes on some firm support. Stand to one side of student in order to get side view of angle formed by trunk and legs when knees are straightened.

Instruction:

Explain the exercise or have some one demonstrate. Caution student to keep hips fixed against stall bars as knees are bent and extended;—do not pull up on arms.

e. AGILITY

1. *Jump*

'Knee chest vault over low boom.' Chapter X. Ex. 7.

Procedure:

Place bar of boom 27–29 inches from floor. Have student stand at one side of it with his side touching it, and grasp it with his hands. The jump is made from two feet, body supported on both hands while knees are bent and brought close to chest as body is swung to opposite side of the bar (still facing same direction). Continue this 6 times, shifting hands (first one in front, then the other), between each jump. Besides clearing the bar, the student should try to make the jump light, keep close to the bar on each side, and use but one jump on each side before crossing.

Instruction:

Explain or demonstrate and let student try it. Have someone near to receive.

2. *Run*

'Back lying' (feet against wall) time.

Procedure:

Have student lie on floor with feet touching the wall, hands at side. Instructor stands 35 feet from student. On signal "go," watch is started and stopped only when student crosses the line 35 feet from starting point.

Instruction:

Caution student to keep up his **momentum** until well past the 35-foot line.

SCORING FOR TESTS

Arm Flexibility

Distance from wall	*Score*
20 inches..........................	9.6–10
18 inches..........................	8.6–9.5
15 inches..........................	7.6–8.5
12 inches..........................	6.6–7.5
10 inches..........................	6 –6.5

Leg Flexibility

Based on ability to bend arms and get trunk **flat against** thighs.

Bar grasped		*Score*
Lowest—	Trunk touching thighs, arms bent, and knees straight, or slightly rounded back.	8.8–10
2nd —	knees straight, back rounded	8 – 8.7
3rd —	knees and arms slightly bent and back rounded, or knees straight, arms straight, and back rounded	7 – 7.9
4th —	arms straight, and back very round	6 – 6.9

Arm Strength

Seconds		*Score*
25	....	10
20–24	....	9
15–19	....	8
10–14	....	7
6– 9	....	6

Leg Strength

Based on ability to keep extended leg straight as bent knee is straightened, body erect, knee bending smooth and rhythmical.

		Score
Straight 6 times	....	8.9–10
Straight 5 times	....	8– 8.8
Straight 4 times	....	7.6– 7.9
Straight 3 times	....	7– 7.5
Straight 2 times	....	6– 6.9

Abdominal Strength

Angle formed by trunk and legs		*Score*
0 degrees or feet touch same bar with hands..........		9.6–10
45– 0 degrees	....	8.9– 9.5
90– 46 degrees	....	8– 8.8
135– 91 degrees	....	7– 7.8
180–134 degrees	....	6– 6.9

Agility

1. Jump—based on lightness, spring and continuous action.

Bar cleared	*Score*
6 times	9.1–10
5 times	8.1– 9
4 times	7.1– 8
3 times	6.1– 7
2 times	0 – 6

2. Run

Time—seconds	*Score*
$3\frac{1}{5}$–3	10
$3\frac{3}{5}$–$3\frac{2}{5}$	9
$4\frac{1}{5}$–$3\frac{4}{5}$	8
$4\frac{3}{5}$–$4\frac{2}{5}$	7
5 –$4\frac{4}{5}$	6

SCORE CHART

FLEXIBILITY	ARM	20 INCHES 10 - 9.6	18 INCHES 9.5 - 8.6	15 INCHES 8.5 - 7.6	12 INCHES 7.5 - 6.6	10 INCHES 6.5 - 6
	LEG	LOWEST BAR 10 - 88	SECOND BAR 8.7 - 8	THIRD BAR 7.9 - 7	FOURTH BAR 6.9 - 6	-
STRENGTH	ARM	25 SECONDS 10	24-20 SECONDS 9	19-15 SECONDS 8	14-10 SECONDS 7	9 SECONDS 6
	LEG	6 TIMES 10 - 8.9	5 TIMES 8.8 - 8	4 TIMES 7.9 - 7.6	3 TIMES 7.5 - 7	2 TIMES 6.9 - 6
	ABD.	10 - 9.6	9.5 - 8.9	88 - 8	7.8 - 7	6.9 - 6
AGILITY	JUMP	6 TIMES 10 - 9.1	5 TIMES 9 - 8.1	4 TIMES 8 - 7.1	3 TIMES 7 - 6.1	2 TIMES 6 -
	RUN	$3-3\frac{1}{5}$ SECONDS 10	$3\frac{2}{5}-3\frac{3}{5}$ SECONDS 9	$3\frac{4}{5}-4\frac{1}{5}$ SECONDS 8	$4\frac{2}{5}-4\frac{3}{5}$ SECONDS 7	$4\frac{4}{5}-5$ SECONDS 6

| | FLEXIBILITY | | | | STRENGTH | | | | | | AGILITY | | | | IND. SCORES | |
| | arm | | leg | | arm | | leg | | abd | | jump | | run | | m | |
	S	M	S	M	S	M	S	M	S	M	S	M	S	M	S	M
A	9	10	9	10	7	10	8	10	7.5	10	9	10	8	10	8.2	10
B	9	10	9	9.8	7	10	6	9	7.5	8.8	7	9	8	8	7.6	9.2
C	8	10	7	9.8	8	8	6.5	10	7	9.5	7	10	8	10	7.4	9.6
D	7	9	6	8.5	8	10	9	9	7	8.8	8	10	8	9	7.6	9.2
E	7	9	7	8.5	9	10	7	10	8	9	7	9.5	9	9	7.7	9.3
F	8	8.8	6	7.5	8	10	8.5	10	7	8.5	9	9.5	8	8	7.8	8.9
G	8	10	7	9.5	6	10	8	8.5	8	9	9	9.5	9	9	7.9	9.4
H	7	8.5	8	9	8	10	7	8.5	6	8.5	7.5	9.5	8	8	7.4	8.9
I	7	8.5	6	9.8	7	10	7.5	10	7.5	10	8.5	10	8	10	7.4	9.8
J	7	10	7	10	10	10	7	10	7.5	9.8	9	10	8	9	7.9	9.8
K	8	9.8	7	8.8	6	10	7	10	7	8.8	7.5	10	9	9	7.4	9.5
L	6.5	9	6.5	8.5	8	10	8	10	8	8.8	6	8.5	9	10	7.4	9.3
M	8	9.5	7.5	9.5	7	10	9	10	7	9.8	9	10	10	10	8.2	9.8
N	10	10	8	10	10	10	9	10	10	10	9.5	10	10	10	9.5	10
m	7.8	9.4	7.2	9.2	7.8	9.9	7.7	9.6	7.5	9.2	8.1	9.7	8.6	9.2	7.8	9.5

Table I—Class chart of recording tests of flexibility, strength and agility scores. Junior Class, C. S. H. P. E., 1926–1927.

Key
- Letters—Names of individuals.
- S —September examination.
- M —May examination.
- m —Class and individual mean.

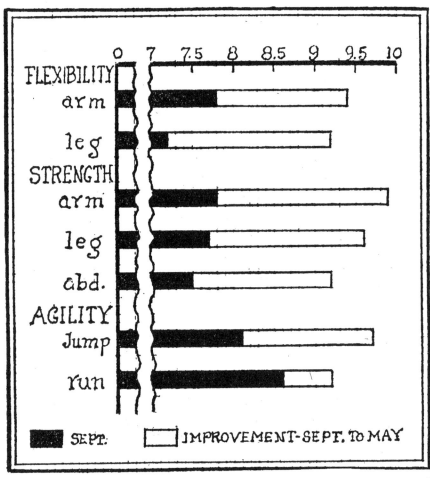

Diagram I. Showing class means in flexibility, strength and agility in September, 1926, and the improvement from September to May, 1927. Junior Class, Central School of Hygiene and Physical Education, New York.

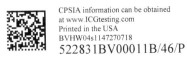

CPSIA information can be obtained
at www.ICGtesting.com
Printed in the USA
BVHW04s1147270718
522831BV00011B/46/P